Medication Management in Older Adults

Susan Koch · F. Michael Gloth
Rhonda Nay
Editors

Medication Management in Older Adults

A Concise Guide for Clinicians

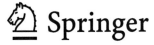 Springer

Editors
Susan Koch
Latrobe University
Division of Nursing and Midwifery
Australia
S.Koch@latrobe.edu.au

Rhonda Nay
Latrobe University
Institute of Social Participation
3552 Bundoora Victoria, Australia
r.nay@latrobe.edu.au

F. Michael Gloth
Johns Hopkins University
School of Medicine
Victory Springs Senior Health
Associates
Business Center Drive 210
21205 Reisterstown Maryland
USA
fgloth1@jhmi.edu

ISBN 978-1-60327-456-2   e-ISBN 978-1-60327-457-9
DOI 10.1007/978-1-60327-457-9
Springer New York Dordrecht Heidelberg London

Library of Congress Control Number: 2010930597

Printed on acid-free paper

Springer is part of Springer Science+Business Media (www.springer.com)

Preface

As medication errors can occur at all stages in the medication process, from prescription by physicians to delivery of medication to the patient by nurses, and in any site in the health system, it is essential that interventions be targeted at all aspects of medication delivery.

Dollars spent on counteracting adverse drug events are dollars unavailable for other purposes. But not all the costs can be directly measured. Errors are also costly in terms of loss of trust in the system by patients and diminished satisfaction by both patients and health professionals. Patients who experience a longer hospital stay or disability as a result of medication errors pay with physical and psychological discomfort. Healthcare professionals pay with loss of morale and frustration at not being able to provide the best care possible.

This book presents available evidence on research interventions designed to reduce the incidence of medication errors. This includes discussion regarding common errors and presents the best available evidence related to the identification and management of medication incidents (errors) associated with the prescribing, dispensing, and administration of medicines to older people in the acute, subacute, and residential (long-term) care settings.

While there may be some overlap in the content, it should be noted that there are some subtle differences in the extent of the information provided and the research available to present.

The chapters cover the principles of medical ethics in relation to medication management; common medication errors in the acute care sector; medication management in long-term care settings; nutrition and medications; the outcomes of a systematic review; dose form alterations; electronic health records (EHR), computerized order entry (COE), and Beers criteria; pharmacokinetics; and pharmacodynamics.

The contributors to the book are from Australia and USA providing you with their inspirations and research findings. We hope you enjoy using this handbook to provide the best possible outcomes for older people in your care.

Bundoora, VIC   Susan Koch
Reisterstown, MD   F. Michael Gloth
Bundoora, VIC   Rhonda Nay

Contents

Contributors

Yvonne Coleman, B App Sci (Fd Sci and Nutn), G Dip Diet, G Dip Hlth Ed & Prom
Nutrition Consultants Australia

Catherine Edgar, SEN, RN, Dip App Sci (Nsg), Grad Dip Neurosciences, MNS
Clinical Nurse Consultant, Bundoora Extended Care Centre

Helen Forbes, PhD, RN
Senior Lecturer, Deakin University

F. Michael Gloth
Division of Geriatric Medicine and Gerontology, Johns Hopkins University School of Medicine, Baltimore, MD, USA

Penny Harvey, MD, MBChB, FRACP
Senior Geriatrician, Northern Health, Melbourne, Australia

Sarah N Hilmer, PhD, FRACP
Associate Professor, Departments of Clinical Pharmacology and Aged Care, University of Sydney and Royal North Shore Hospital, St Leonards, Australia

Brent Hodgkinson, (Grad Cert Health Economics, Grad. Cert. Public Health MSc. Physiology, BSc. Biochemistry Honours)
Senior Research Facilitator, Blue Care Research Fellow, University of Queensland

Sue Hunt, PhD
Senior Advisor, Office of Aged Care Quality and Compliance, Australian Government Department of Health and Ageing

David Le Couteur, PhD, MBBS (Hons I), Grad Cert Ed, FRACP
Professor of Geriatric Medicine, Centre for Education & Research on Ageing, Concord Repatriation General Hospital, Sydney, Australia

Hal Kendig, MA, PhD
Research Professor of Ageing and Health, Faculty of Health Sciences and Centre for Education and Research on Ageing, University of Sydney and Concord RG Hospital

Susan Koch, PhD
Associate Professor, Gerontic Nursing at La Trobe University, Melbourne, Australia
Director of Research and Higher Degrees at the Division of Nursing and
Midwifery La Trobe University and Director (Collaborations) Australian Centre
for Evidence Based (ACEBAC)

Andrew McLachlan, PhD, BPharm, FPS
Professor of Pharmacy (Aged Care), Faculty of Pharmacy, Concord RG Hospital,
Concord Repatriation General Hospital, University of Sydney and the Centre for
Education and Research on Ageing

Michael Murray, MBBS, FRACP, MPH, FAAG
Director of Geriatric Medicine, St Vincent's Health, Melbourne, VIC, Australia
Adjunct Associate Professor, Australian Centre for Evidence Based Aged Care

Vasi Naganathan, PhD, FRACP
Associate Professor, Centre for Education and Research on Ageing,
University of Sydney and Concord RG Hospital

Iqbal Ramzan, DipPharm, CIT NZ, MSc, PhD
Professor of Pharmacy, Faculty of Pharmacy, University of Sydney

Pauline Wong
GradCert Health Informatics, PGDipAdvNsg (ClinNsgEd), CritCareCert, BNurs
(Honors), DipAppSci (Nsg)
Lecturer/Course Coordinator, La Trobe University/The Alfred Clinical
School of Nursing, Melbourne, Australia

Is There a Problem? The Evidence of Types and Causes of Medication Errors by Healthcare Workers

Michael Murray

Keywords Older people • Elderly • Ageing • Medication use • Medication errors • Prescribing

Is There a Problem?

Medication can be defined as a natural or artificial substance or a combination of substances used with the primary intent of treating an illness. Medication use is the common and predominant form of health intervention in our society. As we age, the likelihood of medication use increases: 42% of the population below 15 years of age use medications, while 86% of those above 65 years use one or more medications [1]. Medication use will rise substantially in the next 50 years given that Australia, like much of the rest of the world, is an ageing society. In 2007, 13% of Australia's population was aged over 65; and by 2056, this is estimated to rise to between 23% and 25% [2]. Thus, the potential for a medication-related adverse event, including medication errors, also increases.

While medication errors are likely to occur more commonly in older adults, simply on the basis of the probability of the greater use of medication in this population, do these errors constitute a significant problem? Much alarm and publicity were generated in the past when it was suggested by Lazarou [3] that adverse drug reactions were the sixth leading cause of death in the USA. A review of the meta-analysis by Kvasz [4] suggested significant flaws in the design and therefore the validity of the meta-analysis with substantial differences noted between the included studies, thus raising the issue of overestimation. Ross [5] suggested that the terminology in this area was 'a tower of Babel' with no uniformity in event definition. This communication dilemma highlights the difficulty in comparing

M. Murray (✉)
Geriatric Medicine, St Vincent's, Melbourne, Australia
e-mail: Michael.murray@svhm.org.au

S. Koch et al. (eds.), *Medication Management in Older Adults:
A Concise Guide for Clinicians*, DOI 10.1007/978-1-60327-457-9_1,
© Springer Science+Business Media, LLC 2010

studies from different jurisdictions and evaluating the severity of a problem that most health workers know from their own experience is quite significant.

In an attempt to clarify an area that Nebeker et al. [6] felt was "underappreciated and misunderstood," they provided a clinicians guide to terminology, which sought to clarify the relationship between medication errors, adverse drug reactions and adverse drug events (ADEs). They drew upon sources, including definitions by the WHO and the National Coordinating Council for Medication Error Reporting and Prevention first published in [7]. Nebeker cited evidence (admittedly nearly 10 years old at the time) that suggested that approximately 25% of all ADEs were caused by medication errors.

The National Coordinating Council for Medication Error Reporting and Prevention [7] defines a medication error in the following terms:

'A medication error is any preventable event that may cause or lead to inappropriate medication use or patient harm while the medication is in the control of the health care professional, patient, or consumer'.

Such a definition differs chiefly from an ADE in that it is preventable and may cause harm, whereas an ADE is generally now accepted to be associated with harm. Unfortunately, while definitions have been suggested, their variable application continues to make the assessment of studies difficult.

Medication Errors in the Community

Though attention and headlines are more often focused on hospital care and transition the movement of patients between hospital and their community (and vice versa), most prescribing and most medication incidents are likely to occur in the community and relate to the same potential causative list described above. While much has been written about medication errors, there are relatively few studies upon which one can draw evidence-based conclusions. (For types of medication errors in general practice, see Table 1).

In an Australian study on ADEs in a general practice setting, an ADE was defined as an 'unintended event due to the use of a medication that could have harmed or did harm the patient' [8]. They used a definition that lies somewhere between what is now generally accepted as an ADE and a medication error. In this study, more than 15% of those over 65 years experienced an ADE in the preceding 6 months. While it is likely that this was an underrepresentation, given the retrospective nature of the study, it should be noted that the vast majority of these ADEs were as a result of a recognised side effect (72%) or drug sensitivity (12%) with only a small minority related to what would now be defined as a medication error with the emphasis on preventability [8]. In this general practice-based study, preventable medication errors – particularly those involving healthcare workers – appeared uncommon, with prescribing errors and the prescription of drug or drug combinations with contraindications together making up less than 1%. What is unknown is, however, the issue of aetiology of these apparent medication errors.

Table 1 Types of medication errors in general practice

Types of medication error	Rate per 100 incidents Bhasale et al. [9]	Rate per 100 incidents Gilbert et al. [11]
Use of inappropriate or unnecessary drug	30	17
Need for additional medication		11.6
Prescribing error	22	
Administration error	18	
Dose inappropriate	15	13.1
Side effect	13	8.5
Allergic reaction	11	
Dispensing error	10	
Overdose	8	
System inadequacies	7	
Drug omitted or withheld	6	
Interaction	4	1
Non-compliance	4	5
Medication ceased	3	
Contraindication	3	2

Source: Table parameters adapted from [9, 11]

Table 2 Causative or contributing factor to medication errors in general practice

Contributing factor	Rate per 100 incidents
Poor communication between patient and health professionals	23
Action of others (i.e., not GP or patient)	23
Error of judgement	22
Poor communication between health professionals	19
Patient consulted other medical officer	15
Failure to recognise signs and symptoms	15
Patient's history not adequately reviewed	13
Omission of checking procedure	10
GP tired/rushed/running late	10
Patient misunderstood their problem/treatment	10
Inadequate patient assessment	10
Administrative inadequacies	9

Source: Bhasale et al. [9]

It is unclear whether they represent simple slips, errors of omission or commission or inadequate medical knowledge regarding side effects. Though not addressed in this study, an earlier study of all adverse incidents (including but not limited to ADEs) undertaken by Bhasale et al. [9] suggested that poor doctor–patient communication may have contributed in as many as half of all cases. For a list of causative or contributing factors to medication errors in general practice, (see Table 2).

In Bhasale's study [9], there was a much higher rate of what would appear to be medication errors on the part of a health professional, with the bulk of the 407 pharmacological incidents being both preventable and health professional related, though not all could be determined given the limited information supplied.

Similar errors to those seen in Millers [8] study were evident; however, there was a much greater incidence of prescribing errors (22 per 100 incidents) and dispensing errors with 10 per 100 incidents. One may postulate that the increased use of medical software, including prescription software with its automatic drug interaction alerts, in the years between the two studies may be in part responsible for the dramatic decrease in their errors. Similarly, one may also wonder at the negligible take-up of similar prescriber softwares in the acute health sector, in spite of studies, nearly a decade old, demonstrating improved prescription in inpatient care with decreased medication errors and increased appropriate use of anticoagulation [10]. Of more than a little concern in Bhasale's study [9] was that 17% of the documented incidents resulted in major harm with 4% of the incidents resulting in the death of the patients.

In Gilbert et al.'s [11] study of 1,000 at risk community patients with a median age of 72 for men and 74 for women, patients underwent a community pharmacy review with resultant recommendations discussed with the treating doctor. There were 640 recommendations made to change medication because of what was classified as inappropriate/wrong drug being taken and of these 289 (45%) changes were implemented after consultation with the doctor.

While the study design suggested that hospital-based pharmacists supported the community pharmacists who appeared relatively clinically inexperienced, there was neither evidence of blinding nor of inter-rater reliability being undertaken. No data was provided regarding adverse patient outcome or harm as a result of either current medication management or subsequent intervention. Though not defined as such, it is likely that many of the 'medication problems' identified in the review were in fact potential medication errors; however, given that less than 50% of these were acted upon it is likely that at least some represent appropriate prescription with a balanced risk assessment and not a medication error.

The lack of outcome data particularly related to morbidity, mortality and hospital admissions make estimating the scope of the problem difficult. More recent reviews and meta-analysis [12] have either failed to find evidence that pharmacist-led intervention is effective in reducing mortality or admissions or found at best weak evidence of benefit in the primary care setting [13]. A review by Krska et al. [14] of the documentation and completeness of the drug interaction data used by the pharmacists to develop recommendations demonstrated significant variability in accuracy and completeness, thus perhaps explaining the lack of efficacy in the pharmacist-led interventions.

Roughead and Lexchin [15] suggest that on the basis of Millers study, 138,000 people suffered an ADE and required hospitalisation. Further, some of these side effects may have been anticipated (and thus be potentially preventable) if optimal pharmacovigilance had been undertaken prior to market approval or, at the very least, timely conveyed to the prescriber given that in as many as half of all the new drugs serious adverse effects were detected post-marketing approval. What is less clear, is whether or not this increased knowledge would have dramatically altered the number of medication errors i.e., knowing of a potential new adverse effect would this knowledge have altered prescribing practices? Or resulted in additional warning to the patient regarding both risk and potential adverse side effects? Further would knowledge gained have reduced the severity of adverse outcomes by precipitating an early cessation of the medication or at least a timely a review with a risk and benefit evaluation being undertaken by the treating clinician and patient?

Given that some of the 10% increase in hospital admissions for gastrointestinal bleeds in Ontario have been postulated as linked to the 41% increase in use of Cox2 inhibitors, including rofecoxib over the same period [16], it is likely that if true, medication errors have economic and social/health costs greater than previously estimated with greater responsibility linked to healthcare workers.

Medication Errors in Residential Care

While this topic is discussed in more detail in chapter 'Common Medication Errors in Long Term Care Settings', it should be noted that medication errors have been rarely studied in residential care. It is likely that this frail group of people are both more at risk and less able to tolerate adverse events than other more robust sectors of the community. Residents in residential care or nursing facilities are more dependant on the appropriate, accurate and timely provision of medications with less ability to be an active participant in the therapeutic partnership. Thus, while all the types of medication errors outlined in Table 1 are relevant to the doctor/patient nexus, many of the administration issues seen in hospital care are also of particular importance. The accuracy of drug supply with all its component parts ("order communication; product labelling, packaging and nomenclature; compounding; dispensing"), particularly related to medication dose administration aids (DAAs), is also relevant given the increased dependency of nursing and other care staff on these medication-containing aids.

In a review of medication supply errors in aged care facilities, Carruthers et al. [17] audited DAAs accuracy. There was an incident rate of 4.3% of packs audited involving 12% of residents. Missing drug was the most common error on the part of the pharmacy/supply chain, whereas a failure to communicate a change in medication was the most common error attributable to the doctor. The doctor was implicated in 26% (23% if prescription not supplied was excluded), whereas the pharmacy was implicated in 42%. While the resident outcome with respect to medication errors was beyond the scope of the study cited, it should be noted that Analgesics followed by cardiovascular drugs were the top two classes of drugs involved in errors.

Hansen [18] studied medication errors submitted by nursing homes to the state of North Carolina using the NCCMERP definition over a 9-month period. There were 9,272 errors from 384 homes reported with many of the most commonly involved drugs (CNS agents 16% and analgesics 11%), which are also potentially the most serious. Those facilities with proportionately greater number of errors also had potentially more serious drugs involved in the error and the error was less likely to be identified prior to reaching the patient. Though severity of the outcome was not defined, it is likely that if such findings were generalizable, this would represent a serious problem related to healthcare workers.

It has been postulated that the rate of medication errors increases as the nurse–patient ratio within a given sector falls [19]; however, it is unclear in either of the described studies whether this was a factor. Administration of drugs from impress stock necessitating more senior nursing staff has conversely been suggested to carry a substantially greater risk [20]; thus, it is not simply an issue of the staff seniority alone, rather it is likely to be the interplay of staffing levels, expertise and mode of medication delivery that impact on medication errors.

Medication Errors and Hospital Care

This aspect of medication management is discussed in depth in chapter 'Common Medication Errors in the Acute Care Sector'. Medication errors are common in hospitals. While the NCCMERP-described range of potentially causative events are just as evident, Nichols et al. [21] in reviewing the contributory causes of medication errors over a 6 month period categorised the errors into prescribing, dispensing or administration errors due to slips (lack of attention) or lack of knowledge particularly related to unfamiliar drugs, patients and with policy. See Table 3 for causative or contributing factors to medication errors in hospitals and Table 4 for types of medication errors in hospitals.

While methodological issues make comparison of studies difficult, prescribing errors and administration errors have been cited as the two most common medication errors in hospital [22]. The third major category, dispensing errors are less studied and in probability less common with studies suggesting a rate of between 0.08% and 0.8% [20].

Estimates of prescribing errors range from 2–5% [22] to 2–14% with a median rate of 7% [23] of all medication orders; however, many errors are remediated prior to harm. Of these, dosage errors are the most common [23]. Of special concern have been those prescribing errors associated with transition points in care. Such typical transition points occur with entry into the hospital and are frequently compounded

Table 3 Causative or contributing factor to medication errors in hospital

Contributing factor	Source [21]	Source [31]
Poor communication (%)	25	25
Deficiencies in policy (%)	25	25
Lack of knowledge (%)		18
Lack of guidance (%)	27	
Unfamiliar patients (%)	31	
Unfamiliar ward (%)	19	

Table 4 Types of medication errors in hospitals

Categories of medication error	Site of error	Error types
Prescription errors	Transition points, including admission, discharge and intra hospital transfer Transcribing of drug orders and charts Transcription or recording of drug allergies	Errors of omission Ambiguous or illegible order Incorrect dose Wrong drug Inappropriate or not required drug Wrong dosage Wrong frequency Wrong duration Wrong time Wrong route of administration
Administration errors	Errors relating to medication documentation/drug charts including Recording of activity/failure of Interpretation and misreading of medication Delivery of medications	Wrong patient Incorrect dose/concentration Wrong drug Wrong frequency Wrong time or duration Missed dose Wrong route of administration Provision of non-charted drug
Dispensing errors	Central or ward based dispensing from individualised supply or ward stock/impress Discharge supply	Wrong drug Incorrect directions/labelling Incorrect preparation or compounding Incorrect storage (e.g. temperature, use by date, light exposure)

Source: Table parameters adapted from [22]

by movement between units and streams of care, including admission to the emergency department, transfer to an acute medical or surgical service, transition to a step-down facility or service and ultimately discharge. Tam et al. [24] in reviewing prescribing errors as a result of an incomplete medication history at admissions suggested that between 27% and 54% had at least one error of omission with 11–59% of these errors in the cited studies being clinically important. Omitted medications were not trivial with medications most commonly involved included cardiovascular agents, sedatives and analgesics.

The process of medication reconciliation, usually on the part of the pharmacist wherein the medication chart or admission accuracy is checked against a patient's pre-admission medications (even where that pre-admission maybe from a different acute inpatient unit rather than their usual place of residence), remains in its infancy in most health services and jurisdictions. Similarly, the porosity of therapeutics decision support software that is readily accessible to support medication policy adherence and knowledge enhancement continues to be the exception rather than the rule [25] in spite of emerging evidence to support its utility.

Estimating Harm

Estimating harm i.e., the critical extent of the problem is difficult owing the wide range of definitions of prescribing errors in the literature, never the less a range of 1–3% of inpatients has been quoted in literature reviews [26, 27] and as such would constitute a serious problem in the context of a health service. Extremes of age have been identified as a potential patient risk factor for medication errors in the intensive care setting with the addition of each additional medication increasing risk [28]. Though not studied directly in all ward environments, given that older people constitute a substantial percentage of hospitals on same day admissions and majority of occupied bed days and are frequently on a greater number of medications, the burden of harm is likely to fall disproportionally on that group. If the less critical timing errors were excluded and using an average 10% error rate directly observed in Barker et al.'s [29] study and assuming ten doses per older patient per day (almost certainly a significant underestimate) this would result in each older patient subject to one error per day.

Incomplete reporting appears a significant issue at least in the Australian literature with a minority of doctors and nurses reporting near miss medication errors (<20%) and only 40% of doctors reporting errors that resulted in a patient receiving therapeutic intervention. This is in spite of the belief among doctors and nurses in a cross-sectional survey that errors should be reported [30]. National surveys of patient and doctor attitudes to medical errors suggest that even though many have personal or family experience of medical errors, this was not considered a serious problem [32]. Low reporting rates at least among some health professionals, along with the perception that an error is a lesser health issue and priority, would suggest that the seriousness of the problem is significantly underestimated.

Conclusion

Medication errors are common in all areas of health. Just how common in each jurisdiction remains somewhat unclear, in part related to inadequate reporting, in part to an only slowly emerging consensus on just what we are recording, in part to inadequate research on medication errors and in part to the lack of knowledge regarding the appropriateness of prescribing, particularly in the old often in the absence of evidence-based practice. Harm is clearly occurring through omissions and commissions by healthcare workers. Medications are the major current and foreseeable form of health intervention and given that the older person is both a major user of medication and more dependant on the health professional than any other adult, safe, appropriate and error free prescribing is needed. While we may lack many of the answers and have only partial insight into all the contributing factors it is clear that even when direction through evidence is provided most jurisdictions lack the resolve to act. Roughead and Lexchin's [15] is just as apt for medication errors as it is for all ADEs "counting is not enough, action is needed".

Yes, Houston, we have a problem.

References

1. Australian Bureau of Statistics (1995) National health survey: use of medications, Australia, Cat. no. 4377.0, Canberra, 1999. http://www.abs.gov.au/ausstats/abs@.nsf/productsbytitle/BF 60D2B59D518692CA2568A9001393D1?OpenDocument)
2. Australian Bureau of Statistics (2008) Population projections, Australia, 2006 to 2101. http://www.abs.gov.au/ausstats/abs@.nsf/mf/3222.0?OpenDocument. Accessed 10 Sep 2008
3. Lazarou J, Pomeranz BH, Corey PN (1998) Incidence of adverse drug reactions in hospitalized patients. JAMA 279:1200–1205
4. Kvasz M, Allen IE, Gordon MJ, et al (2000) Adverse drug reactions in hospitalized patients: a critique of a meta-analysis. Med Gen Med. http://www.medscape.com/viewarticle/408052_8
5. Ross SD (2001) Drug-related adverse events: a readers' guide to assessing literature reviews and meta-analyses. Arch Intern Med 161:1041–1046
6. Nebeker J, Barach P, Samore M (2004) Clarifying adverse drug events: a clinician's guide to terminology, documentation, and reporting. Ann Intern Med 140:795–801
7. National Coordinating Council for Medication Error Reporting and Prevention. What is a medication error? (2005) Available at http://www.nccmerp.org/aboutMedErrors.html. Accessed 15 July 2009
8. Miller G, Britt H, Valenti L (2006) Adverse drug events in general practice patients in Australia. Med J Aust 184(7):321–324
9. Bhasale AL, Miller GC, Reid SE, Britt HC (1998) Analysing potential harm in Australian general practice: an incident-monitoring study. Med J Aust 169(2):73–76
10. Kuperman GJ, Teich JM, Gandhi TK, Bates DW (2001) Patient safety and computerized medication ordering at Brigham and Women's Hospital. Jt Comm J Qual Improv 27(10):509–521
11. Gilbert AL, Roughead EE, Beilby J, Mott K, Barratt JD (2002) Collaborative medication management services: improving patient care. Med J Aust 177(4):189–192
12. Holland R, Desborough J, Goodyer L, Hall S, Wright D, Loke YK (2008) Does pharmacist-led medication review help to reduce hospital admissions and deaths in older people? A systematic review and meta-analysis. Br J Clin Pharmacol 65:303–316
13. Royal S, Smeaton L, Avery AJ, Hurwitz B, Sheikh A (2006) Interventions in primary care to reduce medication related adverse events and hospital admissions: systematic review and meta-analysis. Qual Saf Health Care 15:23–31
14. Krska J, Avery AJ, on behalf of The Community Pharmacy Medicines Management Project Evaluation Team (2008) Evaluation of medication reviews conducted by community pharmacists: a quantitative analysis of documented issues and recommendations. Br J Clin Pharmacol 65:386–396
15. Roughead EE, Lexchin J (2006) Adverse drug events: counting is not enough, action is needed. Med J Aust 184(7):315–316
16. Mamdani M, Juurlink DN, Kopp A et al (2004) Gastrointestinal bleeding after the introduction of COX2 inhibitors: ecological study. Br Med J 328:1415–1416
17. Carruthers A, Naughton K, Mallarkey G (2008) Accuracy of packaging of dose administration aids in regional aged care facilities in the Hunter area of New South Wales. Med J Aust 188(5):280–282
18. Hansen RA, Greene SB, Williams CE, Blalock SJ, Crook KD, Akers R et al (2006) Types of medication errors in North Carolina nursing homes: a target for quality improvement. Am J Geriatr Pharmacother 4(1):52–61
19. Garretson S (2004) Nurse to patient ratios in American health care. Nurs Stand 19(14–16):33–37
20. Runciman WB, Roughead EE, Semple SJ et al (2003) Adverse drug events and medication errors in Australia. Int J Qual Health Care 15(Suppl 1):i49–i59
21. Nichols P, Copeland TS, Craib IA, Hopkins P, Bruce DG (2008) Learning from error: identifying contributory causes of medication errors in an Australian hospital. Med J Aust 188(5):276–278

22. Australian Commission on Safety and Quality in Health Care (2008) Windows into safety and quality in health care. ACSQHC, Sydney
23. Lewis PJ, Dornan T, Taylor D, Tully MP, Wass V, Ashcroft DM (2009) Prevalence, incidence and nature of prescribing errors in hospital inpatients: a systematic review. Drug Saf 32(5):379–389
24. Tam V, Knowles S, Cornish P, Fine N, Marchesano R, Etchells E (2005) Frequency, type and clinical importance of medication history errors at admission to hospital: a systematic review. CMAJ 173(5):510–515
25. Hughes C (2008) Medication errors in hospitals: what can be done? Med J Aust 188(5):267–268
26. Franklin B, Vincent C, Schachter M, Barber N (2005) The incidence of prescribing errors in hospital in-patients. Drug Saf 28(10):891–900
27. McCarter T, Centafont R, Daly F, Kokoricha T, Leander J (2003) Reducing medication errors a regional approach for hospitals. Drug Saf 26(13):937–950
28. Camiré E, Moyen E, Stelfox H (2009) Medication errors in critical care: risk factors, prevention and disclosure. CMAJ 180(9):936–943
29. Barker KN, Flynn EA, Pepper GA, Bates DW, Mikeal RL (2002) Medication errors observed in 36 health care facilities. Arch Intern Med 162:1897–1903
30. Evans SM, Berry JG, Smith BJ et al (2006) Attitudes and barriers to incident reporting: a collaborative hospital study. Qual Saf Health Care 15:39–43
31. NSW Health (2006) Patient safety and clinical quality program. Third report on incident management in the NSW public health system 2005–2006, Sydney, NSW Health. http://www.health.nsw.gov.au/pubs/2006/patient_safety_3.html. Accessed July 2009
32. Blendon RJ, DesRoches CM, Brode CM et al. (2002) Views of practicing physicians and the public on medical errors. N Engl J Med 24:1933–1940

Quality Use of Medicines: Policy and Practice

Susan Hunt

Keywords Quality use of medicines • Consumer medicines information • Medication management guidelines • National Prescribing Service • Drug use evaluation • Policy

Introduction

The problems related to the use of medicines by older people are often described in terms of adverse drug events or misadventures. However, medicines have done much to increase the overall well-being of older people by treating chronic diseases, alleviating pain and contributing to the quality of life [1]. Policies to influence medication use have varied among countries according to historical, political and funding factors. While the health systems of countries vary markedly, the need for strategies which support quality use of medicines (QUM) by older people is similar. QUM has enabled clinicians to move to a position where they can work *with* older people to use medicines more wisely.

This chapter explores the QUM policy development and some of the practice strategies which support the QUM by older people.

Setting the Scene for QUM Policy Development

Following the World War II, the supply of affordable medicines became a global concern and, therefore, a preoccupation of governments. The United Kingdom (UK) included the supply of medicines as part of the National Health System (NHS), while in the United States of America (USA), the supply and payment of

S. Hunt (✉)
Office of Aged Care Quality and Compliance,
Australian Government Department of Health and Ageing
e-mail: susan.hunt@health.gov.au

S. Koch et al. (eds.), *Medication Management in Older Adults:*
A Concise Guide for Clinicians, DOI 10.1007/978-1-60327-457-9_2,
© Springer Science+Business Media, LLC 2010

medicines varies from state to state, with a mix of government initiatives, third party or insurance schemes and largely, consumer payments [2]. Canada has developed a number of initiatives to ensure access to essential medicines, which vary among provinces.

The Australian government's response to the challenge of ensuring Australians access to affordable and necessary medicines was the development in 1950 of the Pharmaceutical Benefits Scheme (PBS), a scheme that is unique to Australia. By ensuring access to medicines, the formation of the PBS contributed to the health of the Australian population and thereby maximise Australia's ability to contribute to the postwar rebuilding that was necessary in all aspects of the Australian economy [3]. As a result of the formation of the PBS, the life expectancy and health outcomes for many Australians are considered to have been transformed [4].

Access to essential medicines through the PBS is considered a success storey. By 1989, there was increasing evidence that medicines were part of the everyday life for most Australians. The *Australian Health Survey 1989–1990* showed 76% of women and 65% of men had used prescribed and/or over-the-counter (OTC) medicines in the 2 weeks preceding the survey [5]. However, during the mid to late 1980s, there was increasing recognition that although medicines played an important role in protecting, maintaining and restoring health, this role was limited. There was recognition that medication could not be a remedy for the social issues often faced by older people such as loneliness, social isolation or poverty. In addition, for many people, the burden of a medication regimen, both in terms of side effects and cost, can potentially outweigh the beneficial effects of treatment [6, 7].

During the 1980s and 1990s, there was increasing concern over the health, social and economic costs to Australia associated with an inappropriate use of both prescribed and OTC medicines [5]. This was thought to be compounded by both the consumers' attitudes to medicines and the attitudes of those who prescribe [8], and was reinforced by the skilful marketing of the pharmaceutical industry by which a 'pill for every ill' mentality had been encouraged [9]. It was this social mix that framed medicine policy development in Australia. However, policy development in any area rarely has one single driver. Drivers for change for QUM were the economic reality of medicines usage coupled with the health consequences of usage.

Economic consequences of the PBS were and remain a strong driver for policy development around medicines. In 1963, pharmaceuticals formed the largest single item of expenditure under the national health benefits; with the cost rising significantly in the 1970s and 1980s. In 1989/1990, 105 million prescriptions were subsidised under the PBS at a cost of $1.2 billion [4]. In 2006, 237 million prescriptions were dispensed accounting for over 14% ($A3.0 billion) of the recurrent health expenditure [10]. This does not include the amount spent on drugs supplied in public hospitals, or through the Repartition Benefits Scheme (RBS) mainly to service veterans (15 million prescriptions [10]), or through private prescriptions (~54 million prescriptions [10]), or OTC and complementary medicines (CMs).

Cost containment of the pharmaceutical budget however was not the only impetus for policy development. While it was recognised that medicines make a significant contribution to the treatment and prevention of disease and are able to increase life expectancy and improve quality of life, there was increasing evidence that the usage of medicines was less than optimum with consequential poor health outcomes and a resultant increase in the cost of healthcare services. Older people were noted as being particularly at risk of experiencing hospitalisation due to their medication regimens [11].

A systematic review of studies assessing drug-related hospital admissions in Australia indicated that approximately 81,000 hospital admissions in Australia in 1994–1995 were medicine-related [12]. The authors estimated that between 32 and 69% of all medicines-related admissions were considered 'definitely' or 'possibly' preventable. By 2002, it was estimated that around 140,000 hospital admissions each year are associated with problems in the use of medicines among older people, particularly those living in an institution, being at risk [13]. During this time, research showed significant problems with medication usage in long-term care.

Of particular interest to the development of QUM was the increasing criticism about a number of areas of drug usage and older people; for example, poor analgesia use for pain management [5, 14–16], inappropriate antibiotic usage [5, 17] and the lack of treatment of depression experienced by older people [18, 19].

As the QUM policy development was gaining momentum, there were a number of assertions that prescribing of drugs for behaviour control, or chemical restraint, in long-term care was high or inappropriate [18, 20–23]. There was also criticism of the use of antipsychotic drugs with the elderly, with the comment that the use of such medicines as contributing to polypharmacy [24], with potential negative health outcomes such as an increased incidence of falls and/or urinary incontinence [25, 26] and contributing to cognitive impairment including delirium [27, 28]. The issues identified for older people included *over-prescription* of some medication classes, for example benzodiazepines; *under-prescription*, for example of asthma medication; as well as *inappropriate choice* of medicines, for example inappropriate forms of analgesia [29].

QUM Policy Development

Policy development of QUM and the later *National Medicines Policy 2000* (NMP) in Australia involved 'not a single decision, but a web of decisions that [took] place and evolve[d] overtime' [30]. QUM is about a reform of how medicines are used which recognises the complexity of medicine usage. A number of interests are involved; health professional groups particularly pharmacy and medical practitioners, the pharmaceutical manufacturing industry, policy makers as well as consumers [31]. The formulation of a medicines policy involved.

> the realisation that drugs are more than chemical or biological substances with medicinal properties. Drugs are also highly profitable commodities to be researched, patented, marketed and sold. In addition, they are powerful symbols of magic, medicine, professional power, human compassion and political concern [4].

From the late 1970s, through to the early 1990s, there was increasing questioning in the literature as to the place of medicines in the promotion of health; this questioning is an ongoing critique. Social scientists began to look into the production, distribution and consumption of pharmaceuticals. The disciplines of sociology and anthropology contributed to the debates with research exploring the cultural 'meanings' of medicines for people. For example: examining medicines as a dimension of overall health practices [32]; the value placed on certain members of society as 'knowledgeable' and the gendered roles of women as mothers and carers in relation to medicines [33]; the use of western medicines in developing countries [34]; the symbolic meanings attributed to medicines in varying contexts [35, 36]. Rather than viewing medicine usage as 'irrational', this body of knowledge has enabled an understanding of the reasoned basis that underlies people's use of medicines.

In addition, research into the political economy of the production and distribution of western pharmaceuticals [37, 38], and a sociological critique of the cultural and conceptual underpinnings of the pharmaceutical industry and the different interests within it [39] have contributed to the understanding of medicines as a commodity, and the potential role medicines may play in the 'medicalisation' of non-medical problems [40]. There emerged an understanding of the complex and interactive relationship between the pharmaceutical industry and the wider culture as an evolving entity. As pharmaceutical companies aggressively promoted illness and their products to the health professions and the wider community [4], concern was expressed of the emergence of medicalisation of people's social issues [41].

Australia was not alone in experiencing these issues; the need, use and marketing of medicines areinternational concerns. A defining moment for change came in 1985 with a conference of experts convened by the World Health Organisation (WHO). Their deliberations, entitled *The Rational Use of Drugs* [37] were adopted as a resolution by the 39th World Health Assembly in 1986; the resolution urged member states to develop and implement comprehensive drug policies, which the WHO considered essential for addressing the problems that many countries faced in the supply and use of medicines. However, many countries did not, and may still not, have good access to affordable drugs, or access to the right drugs at the right time. The cost to individuals of essential medicines was a problem in a number of countries. For Australia and other developed countries, access to medicines had largely been addressed by various schemes, such as the PBS in Australia, however, the WHO statement was considered to have an important message for those countries where access to essential medicines had been largely solved and where usage might not be optimum:

> Rational use of drugs demands that the appropriate drug be prescribed, that it be available at the right time at a price people can afford, that it be dispensed correctly, and taken at the right dose at the right intervals and for the right length of time. The appropriate drug must be effective, and of acceptable quality and safety… The formulation and implementation by governments of a national drug policy are fundamental to ensure rational drug use [37].

The concerns expressed on the world stage and in research circles came at the time when there was increasing concerns expressed by consumer groups in Australia about the usage of medicines. During the 1970s and 1980s, there were changes in consumer attitudes and expectations with increasing demands for accountability in relation to the services provided by health professionals and, in particular, the inappropriate prescribing of medicines. By the end of the 1980s, this concern 'took on a more articulate form' [42]. For example, the feminist groups were encouraging women to resist the use of benzodiazepines with campaigns using themes such as 'Give Your Feelings a Better Chance: Try to Avoid Tranquillisers' [5], and a collation between the Australian Consumers' Association and the Combined Pensioners' Association developed a teaching resource for use by groups of older people to educate themselves about what to ask of a prescriber or a pharmacist dispensing medicines [43].

Older people had begun to be highly organised and active in demanding better provision of overall healthcare [6]. The Australian Consumers' Association, the Combined Pensioners' Association and the Australian Council on the Ageing (now known as Council on the Ageing) were highly organised groups who undertook their own research into older peoples' experience with medicines [43, 44]; research which has been attributed to being the trigger for both national action and education initiatives [42].

The establishment of the Consumers' Health Forum (CHF) in the mid-1980s, a coalition of many types of health interest groups in Australia, was pivotal. One of its earliest priorities was to improve pharmaceutical policy [45]. Stimulated by the WHO's statement on rational drug use, CHF drafted a discussion document *Towards a national medicinal drug policy for Australia* [46], which was circulated for comment to key stakeholders such as Commonwealth, State and Territory governments, representative organisations of pharmacists, medical practitioners, the pharmaceutical industry, clinical pharmacologists, alcohol and drug societies as well as patient support groups [47]. CHF has continued to investigate and represent consumers' views and experiences with medicines as well as their potential problems with long term drug use, particularly in the management of chronic disease. All of the publications of CHF are available from http://www.chf.org.au; these reports provide a useful resource for anyone wishing to understand the problems experienced by consumers and their wish for change.

The various lobbying resulted in the formation in 1991 of two cross-sectoral committees with the express task of advising the Federal Minister of Health and the relevant federal government department about medicines. Both committees have had a lead role in the formation of medicinal policies, particularly QUM. Known by their acronyms, APAC (Australian Pharmaceutical Advisory Council) and PHARM (Pharmaceutical Health and Rational use of Medicines) had different but complementary agendas.

PHARM's agenda 'was to develop a QUM policy, to develop educational strategies, to assist with funding research projects, and to evaluate issues to do specifically with the way medicines are used' [42]. The inclusive nature of the membership of PHARM was unique; "this was the first time nurses, consumers, and industry were around the table with the 'traditional' multidisciplinary technical expert group of advisers and researchers" [42]. The traditional experts and researchers referred to are doctors, community pharmacists and clinical pharmacologists.

APAC was created as a consultative forum to advise the Australian government on a wide range of pharmaceutical policy issues. APAC was responsible for advice across the whole area of national medicinal drug policy and in this role, could 'comment on, review, or endorse guidelines, standards and practices' [48]. APAC's remit, therefore, was much broader than that of PHARM.

While health professionals and consumer activists were influencing policy development, so too was the Australian government. In 1992, several reports were released, just as PHARM and APAC were developing their first strategic plans. Consequently, these reports have proved highly influential in the subsequent form of the QUM policy and the strategies that have been adopted for its implementation. For example, a three part report from the House of Representatives (federal government) Standing Committee of Community Affairs (HRSCCA) on prescribed health advocated a team approach to the issues related to medication usage [49]. The concept that QUM required a team approach was included in the QUM policy.

Equally influential to the content of the QUM policy was the need for a systems approach to the problems which was advocated by the National Health Strategy (NHS) report (known as the Macklin Report) entitled *Issues in Pharmaceutical Drug Use in Australia*, with 'measures needed to be directed both at the different stages of drug use… and at the multiple organisations and individuals involved in making decisions about drug use' [11]. The Macklin Report concentrated on the consequences of drug use, including deaths and hospital admissions. Among its recommendations to reduce adverse consequences of drug use was the establishment of a national pharmaceutical education programme to provide information to health professionals, consumers and carers on issues related to medicine usage, with the aim to improve the prescribing, dispensing, administration and use of medicines. This recommendation came to fruition in 1998 with the formation of the National Prescribing Service (NPS), the activities of which will be explored later in this chapter.

Developing Solutions: The QUM Approach

It was clear that a uni-level approach to improving medicine usage in Australia was not going to bring about the changes required nor would it have been acceptable to the various players; there was a complex range of 'issues including behavioural, social and political factors which would need to be addressed to improve the use of medicines' [47]. It could be argued that, if health professionals, particularly medical practitioners prescribed more carefully, many of the problems experienced by consumers would not occur. However, the QUM approach sought to move beyond this simplistic approach to involve everyone who prescribed, dispensed, administered or used medicines or considered using medicines.

The goal of QUM was identified as 'to optimise medicinal drug use (both prescription and OTC) to improve health outcomes for all Australians' [5]. The challenge was to develop a theoretical framework which acknowledged the various

The Quality Use of Medicines Pyramid

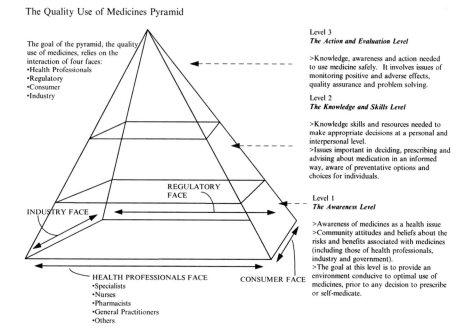

The goal of the pyramid, the quality use of medicines, relies on the interaction of four faces:
•Health Professionals
•Regulatory
•Consumer
•Industry

REGULATORY FACE

INDUSTRY FACE

HEALTH PROFESSIONALS FACE
•Specialists
•Nurses
•Pharmacists
•General Practitioners
•Others

CONSUMER FACE

Level 3
The Action and Evaluation Level

>Knowledge, awareness and action needed to use medicine safely. It involves issues of monitoring positive and adverse effects, quality assurance and problem solving.

Level 2
The Knowledge and Skills Level

>Knowledge skills and resources needed to make appropriate decisions at a personal and interpersonal level.
>Issues important in deciding, prescribing and advising about medication in an informed way, aware of preventative options and choices for individuals.

Level 1
The Awareness Level

>Awareness of medicines as a health issue
>Community attitudes and beliefs about the risks and benefits associated with medicines (including those of health professionals, industry and government).
>The goal at this level is to provide an environment conducive to optimal use of medicines, prior to any decision to prescribe or self-medicate.

Fig. 1 The quality use of medicines pyramid (source: Department of Health Housing and Community Services (1992) A policy of the quality use of medicines. AusInfo, Canberra, p. 18)

players, encouraged cooperation and a partnership approach, facilitated integration of ideas which enabled sustainable change. The result was the QUM pyramid, illustrated in Fig. 1. Each face of the pyramid represents one of the major stakeholders – health professionals, consumers, government and the pharmaceutical industry. Each level of the pyramid represents the stages of learning about medicines, beginning with awareness, moving to development of appropriate knowledge and skills, with the third level being concerned with action and evaluation [50].

Inherent in the QUM framework are the concepts of transferability, of developing knowledge and skills and of sustainability. How these concepts might be facilitated in a number of specific service delivery arenas is yet unknown; however, the intention is to build capacity in the identified players. This is illustrated by the two strategies identified in the QUM policy. The first was the education of all groups identified within the policy, with education defined as 'providing people with the tools of increased awareness, knowledge and information, skills, resources and motivation to take actions that are successful and satisfying' [5]. This was to be coupled with a second strategy of the 'creation of an environment conducive to people making decisions and taking actions that will optimise the QUM', which it was explained as being 'the identification, analysis and investigation of options to overcome structural and other operating constraints affecting the way people live and work' [5].

In summary, the development of the QUM policy is an example of policy development, which involved a number of players each with their own perspectives. However, policy development is not static; through the 1990s, there were a number of voices seeking integration of the QUM policy with other medicinal policies. The launch of the *National Medicines Policy* [51] in December 1999 was the result of this pressure, locating QUM firmly in the wider health policies, and within industry and trade policies.

Developing Integration: National Medicines Policy

In 1999, QUM, instead of being a separate policy, became a strategy in the broader national medicines policy. The result of this was to bring the various dimensions of Australian medicinal policy together for the first time. In addition to QUM, the NMP covered equity of access to affordable medicines and the supply of medicines that met appropriate standards of quality, safety and efficacy with the need for a viable medicines industry. The aim of the NMP is also broader than the promotion of health and includes the dimension of economics: 'the policy aims to meet the medication and related service needs, so that both optimal health outcomes and economic objectives are achieved for Australians' [52].

The reasons underpinning this change have yet to be articulated in the health policy literature. However, at the time the NMP was launched, there was a wider national debate concerning the value to society of expensive treatments and the need to measure, in some way, cost effectiveness in relation to health outcomes. Also at this time, there was an increasing call for both healthcare provision and health policy development to be based on evidence [53]. There was mounting pressure for transparency, accountability and efficiency in all areas of public policy which, in turn, reinforced the demand for evidence. In the NMP, there is the recognition that medicine supply and usage is part of the broader health policies and cannot be viewed separate from the policies covering industry and trade. As shown in Fig. 2, the consumer is considered central to the process.

The overall development of a national medicinal policy has been relatively slow, with the various parts of the policy being developed at different times as a result of varying economic and political imperatives. In addition to the QUM strategy, the other components of the NMP include: equity of access to affordable medicines, which has been achieved through the development of the PBS; a viable Australian pharmaceutical industry which has been achieved through financial incentives to the pharmaceutical industry; and the supply of medicines of acceptable safety, quality and efficacy, which has been achieved through legislation. It is clear that the supply and use of medicines is not simple; a complexity of social and political factors can be identified in the development of QUM as a part of health policy development.

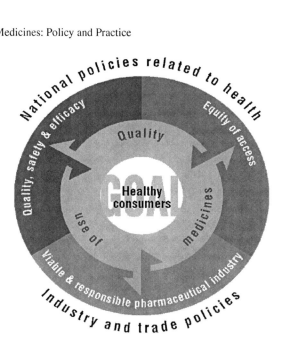

Fig. 2 QUM and the National Medicines Policy (source: Department of Health and Ageing (2002)/ The National Strategy for quality use of medicines. Executive summary. AusInfo, Canberra, p. 2)

QUM in Practice

For people to achieve QUM, they must have the knowledge and skills to use the medicines to their best effect. Important practice initiatives which have been found to support QUM are structures and processes which keep the centrality of the consumer to the medication process, along with strategies which encourage an informed consumer as well as an informed health professional. These include the development of the NPS as an independent source of evidenced-based information about medicines particularly affecting older people, for both health professionals and consumers; and the development of drug usage evaluation (DUE) specifically for long-term care; and the development of guidelines for medication management across the continuum of care.

Evidence-Based Information: The NPS

In an era when there is more information available in more forms than ever before, countries have found it necessary to develop a single source of information about medicines, which can be relied on by both consumers and health professionals. There are issues related to having up-to-date information to aid decision making – this information needs to be independent of pharmaceutical manufacturing marketing as well as free from the perception of government control. The availability of independent, accurate and reliable information, in forms that consumers or health professionals can use, is fundamental to QUM. Countries around the world have solved this problem in a variety of ways. For example, the U.S. Food and Drug Administration (http://www.fda.gov/) has a comprehensive website with specific resources for consumers as well as health professionals.

Two of the fundamental principles of QUM are cooperation and coordination, and support for strategies that have been found to be conducive to QUM. While QUM had been a policy initiative since 1991, by 1997 it was clear that, unless an organisation was given the responsibility for implementing QUM, nothing fundamentally would change. From 1991 until 1997, multiple QUM projects and studies had been funded, but there was no coordinated way to translate successful projects into ongoing programmes and strategies; what was needed was a structure that could assist health professionals and consumers understand what had been found to promote QUM.

Following a national consultation process, the Australian government announced in the 1997–1998 budget funding for a national organisation, the NPS, to undertake work in QUM. The NPS is a public company with an independent board of management and operates within the framework of the National Medicines Policy. The acceptance of NPS has largely been due to it being independent of both government and the pharmaceutical industry. The NPS aims to draw together the expertise of all those involved in medication usage – consumers, pharmacists, hospitals and other institutions, and those who work in them, including community based agencies such as nursing services, the pharmaceutical industry, the government, and of course all prescribers within the medical and other professions.

What NPS has achieved is a central point for evidence-based information about medicines, how they are used and what has been found to support QUM. Fundamental to the work of NPS is the promotion of an informed consumer as well as an informed health professional. Specific consumer campaigns include *Common colds need common sense, not antibiotics* and *Generic medicines are an equal choice* (http://www.nps.org.au); the materials developed including the consumer messages, have universal application.

An Informed Consumer: Consumer Medicines Information (CMI)

The promotion of health and wellbeing is what consumers want from treatment, with accessible and relevant information about their medicines repeatedly being shown as a high priority [54, 55]. It is not only prescribed medicines that are thought to result in an increase risk when used without an understanding of their potential for benefit and harm. With the increasing use of CMs, there has been concern that consumers do not always understand the action, risk of side effects, or the potential for drug–drug or drug–food interactions that can result from the CMs.

Worldwide, consumers purchase a wide range of CMs and consult a range of complementary and alternative medicine practitioners, who may also directly supply CMs. In 2003, an Expert Committee on Complementary Medicines in the Health System was commissioned to report on the status of CMs and therapies in Australia. Their report *Complementary Medicines in the Australian Health System* [56] identified consumers and health professionals have a need for accurate, reliable and independent information about CMs to facilitate safe, appropriate and effective use of CMs, and to allow them to make informed decisions.

While the term 'consumer' does not have universal acceptance in the literature for older people receiving care, it is 'the preferred term of the organised consumer movement in Australia for health service recipients' [57]. As Wade points out 'the term correctly reflects that people in receipt of health care consume services and products provided by others' [57]. An informed consumer can more adequately represent their own wishes to healthcare providers and participate more fully in the care decision processes. There is an expectation in QUM that the consumer, who is central to QUM, will be an active partner in decisions related to their medication therapy [52]. Within QUM, an uninformed person cannot be an active partner in care decisions.

One of the cornerstones of QUM is ensuring that consumers have sufficient information to enable them to use medicines safely and to make informed decisions about their own medication regimens. Accordingly, it is mandatory for all medicines registered for the Australian market after January 1993 to have a CMI leaflet, which is prepared by the pharmaceutical manufacturer and provided by pharmacists at the point of dispensing a medicine. CMI are also available on the web (http://www.nps.org.au). The content of a CMI, written in non-technical language, includes an outline of the benefits, possible side effects of the medicine and how to use the medicine for best effect.

Other countries have also developed similar consumer information about medicines. What is now required is for health professionals to encourage consumers to use this information as part of their decision making about their medication regimens, and thus increase the number of knowledgeable consumers. This is particularly relevant to community dwelling older people, who, with the increased use of medicines as part of the treatment for chronic disease, often have complex medication regimens which may not be well supervised.

Not all older people are community dwellers; many reside in long-term care. Like other countries, the residents of Australian long-term facilities are older, frailer with more chronic ill health than previously [58]. The perception that residents of long-term care do not require information about their medication regimens may be held by health professionals, who believe the degree of frailty of many residents precludes their active involvement in care decisions. However, many residents have family members who are active in care decisions, and who need relevant information written in an easily accessible manner. Some resident have specific advocates that have been identified to speak on their behalf, or a trusted person who holds enduring power of attorney; research has shown a potential role for CMI to enable these people to make informed decisions on behalf of the resident and a willingness of nurses and caregivers working in long-term care to use CMIs as part of their resident and family care planning activities [50].

An Informed Health Professional

With the large number of prescriptions dispensed in Australia, plus an unknown and unquantifiable use of OTC and CMs, it is difficult to know exactly how many people are affected by an adverse drug event, for example, many adverse drug reactions (ADR) are not recognised or reported. There is evidence in the literature that as many as 1 in 12 community-based older people, either through their general practitioner or a hospital outpatient department, may be prescribed inappropriate or wrong drugs [59]. Prescribing for older people is not an exact science; it is a difficult process with many distracters that can lead a prescriber astray.

Helping health professionals keep abreast with the contemporary practices of medicine usage has been one of the challenges in QUM. What has been shown is that multiple forms of information are required, paper-based as well as electronic, with electronic versions that are easily downloadable being increasingly acceptable. For example, *NPS RADAR*, available on the NPS website (http://www.nps.org.au) aims to give health professionals evidence-based information about new drugs, to enable them to assess how a new drug might fit with their current treatment choices; understand how the drug compares with existing therapies; be aware of any key issues when prescribing new drugs; and assess recent published clinical research that may strongly influence the choice and use of the medicines. Downloadable from the internet, health professionals can register for an electronic notification for when a RADAR has been published.

Also available through the NPS website are a number of evidence-based publications, and educational activities such as case studies, clinical audits and pharmacy practice reviews to improve QUM in practice. Many of the therapeutic topics are specific to older people, for example, drug treatment and dementia. The management of medicines in long term has been noted to be highly problematic – there is a shortage of qualified staff in long-term care facilities, as well as residents with complex medication regimens. Older people living in a residential aged care facility are by definition, particularly vulnerable for experiencing a medication misadventure.

DUE is a quality improvement activity, which uses an ongoing cyclical process to improve QUM and health outcomes of residents. It involves monitoring and reviewing drug use, evaluating and comparing it with evidenced-based practice guidelines, and using interventions to improve drug use and overall resident care – this cycle is repeated as often as necessary to achieve the goals decided by the team. Undertaking a DUE has been shown to influence the behaviour of the health professionals undertaking the activity; essentially it can expose taken-for-granted medicines practices. A DUE can bring about a change in actual medicine usage by affecting either the behaviour of the prescriber or those who administer medicines, particularly prn (or whenever necessary) medicines.

The available DUE activities focus on specific disease states or therapeutic areas for residential aged care facilities: examples are antipsychotic use in the management of dementia; benzodiazepine and non-benzodiazepine hypnotics for insomnia; analgesic use for persistent pain; and laxative use for chronic constipation.

The DUE programmes are recognised by a number of health professional bodies as contributing to continuing education and professional development points are awarded on completion.

Development of Medication Management Guidelines

The majority of older people live active, productive lives in their communities. However, due to the numbers of people experiencing chronic ill health with the possibility of hospitalisation, the average age of the patients of acute care facilities is increasing – as a student once commented *old people are everywhere*. There is recognition that, if QUM is to be achieved for older people, it is necessary to acknowledge that older people move between health services as health issues arise; these might be primary care services, tertiary care services, community-based or inpatient, or a mix of all at any one time. An episode of care delivery can be very short, perhaps a matter of hours through to service provision of an extensive period of time. Accordingly, the development of medication management guidelines across the continuum of care was thought to be a necessary QUM practice initiative.

The first of these guidelines covered residential aged care, with the first edition released in 1997 [60], and revised in 2000 and 2002. These guidelines were developed by representatives of the major stakeholder groups, in particular, those representing general practitioners, community pharmacists, nursing and major consumer advocacy groups. In addition, major 'players' in the residential aged care industry were invited to participate. These included representatives of the church and charitable groups plus one of the large for-profit providers. The final edition has 14 recommendations to improve the medication management in residential aged care, and therefore, contribute to QUM for residents; the formation of a medication advisory committee in each facility; what a medication chart should have; the need for regular medication review; medicines should be administered by appropriately trained personnel; the inappropriateness of standing orders in long-term care; nurse-initiation of medicines; self-administration by residents; alteration of dose formulation (more usually called crushing); the use of dose administration aids; the use of information sources for resident and caregivers; how medicines should be stored; the disposal of unwanted medicines; the use of complementary, alternative and self-selected medicines; and the supply of emergency medicines [61].

While it cannot be claimed that the guidelines for medication management in residential aged care solved all of the problems related to managing medicines in long-term care, these guidelines provided a much needed framework to enable caregivers in long-term care to review their medication related practices. Attention then turned to the needs of people, particularly older people, who entered acute care services. There was an evident need for good discharge planning to enable an older person to leave acute care, usually transferring to service providers of primary care, in such a way that continuity of medication was achieved. However, it was clear that a set of guidelines similar to those developed for residential aged care would not be acceptable to the various organisations that provide acute care services, community or primary care; there was a great deal of variability in what constituted good discharge or transfer of a consumer from one service to another. Consequently, in 2005, a set of guiding principles was developed to enable each service to develop protocols, to be used as a basis for the development of operational standards of practice, and to enable each service define performance standards and guidelines for all the medication management activities.

Taking a partnership approach where collaboration and consultation were necessary activities and reflective of QUM, the ten principles held the consumer as central to all medication processes. These principles included the need for healthcare service managers and healthcare professionals to provide leadership to ensure that system exits and resources are provided to enable medication management across the continuum of care; that healthcare service managers and health professionals have a responsibility to participate in all aspects of medication management in partnership with consumers; healthcare service managers and health professionals are jointly and individually accountable for making sure that the activities which support the continuity of medication management are implemented; an accurate and complete medication history should be obtained and documented at the time of admission to care; throughout each episode of care medicines and other therapies should be assessed to ensure QUM; a medication action plan should be developed with the consumer and relevant health professionals which forms an integral part of care planning and which is reviewed before transfer; before transfer to another service, consumers and/or their carers, should have sufficient information in a form they understand to enable the safe and effective use of medicines in accordance with the agreed medication action plan; consumers and their carers should receive sufficient supplies of labelled medicines to enable them to continue treatment whilst transferring to another health service; when a consumer transfers to another care provider, complete and accurate information should be provided to enable continuity of medication management; and the transferring healthcare provider is responsible for evaluating the extent to which continuity of a consumer's medication management has been achieved [62].

The use of these guidelines has yet to be evaluated. However they have proved useful to organisations wishing to move to QUM and the promotion of positive health outcomes for consumers of their services. All of these documents are available from http://www.health.gov.au/ following the links through to all APAC publications.

Conclusion

A number of interests can be identified in the history of the policy development: in particular, the consumer movement which was highly influential in the early stages, the pharmacy and medical professions, the pharmaceutical industry and the governments.

QUM provides a framework to view medicines with the consumers as central to all medication related processes. What constitutes QUM in varying service settings is yet to be fully explored; however, a number of practice initiatives have been developed to enable healthcare professionals and consumers to become active partners in QUM.

References

1. Hunt S (2007) Older adulthood. In: Crisp J, Taylor C (eds) Potter & Perry's fundamentals of nursing, 3rd edn. Elsevier, Sydney, pp 239–266
2. Hughes CM, Roughhead E, Kerse N (2008) Improving use of medicines for older people in long-term care: contrasting the policy approach of four countries. Health Policy 3(3):1–14
3. Sloan C (1995) A history of the pharmaceutical benefits scheme 1947–1992. Commonwealth Department of Human Services and Health, Canberra
4. Harvey K, Murray M (1995) Medicinal drug policy. In: Gardner H (ed) The politics of health. Churchill Livingstone, Melbourne, pp 238–283
5. Department of Health Housing and Community Services (1992) A policy on the quality use of medicines. Department of Health, Housing and Community Services, Canberra, in conjunction with the Pharmaceutical Health and the Rational use of Medicines (PHARM) Working Party
6. Australian Council on the Ageing (1990) Conference panel presentations and recommendations. Medications and older people: addressing the issues. ACOTA, Melbourne
7. Consumers' Health Forum (1999) Easing the burden – the pharmaceutical benefits scheme and people with chronic conditions. Consumers' Health Forum of Australia, Canberra
8. Cockburn J, Pitt S (1997) Prescribing behaviour in clinical practice: patients' expectations and doctors 'perceptions of patients' expectations – a questionnaire study. Br Med J 315:520–523
9. Brudon-Jacobowicz P (1994) From research to practice: bridging the gap. In: Etkin NL, Tan ML (eds) Medicines: meanings & contexts. Health Action Information Network and Medical Anthropology Unit, University of Amsterdam, Amsterdam, pp 9–14
10. Australian Institute of Health and Welfare (2008) Australia's health 2008. AIHW cat. no. AUS 99. Australian Institute of Health and Welfare, Canberra
11. Macklin J (1992) Issues in pharmaceutical drug use in Australia, Issues paper no. 4. National Health Strategy, Department of Health, Housing and Community Services, Canberra
12. Roughead E, Gilbert AL, Primrose JG, Sanson LN (1998) Drug-related hospital admissions: a review of Australian studies published 1988–1996. Med J Aust 168:405–408
13. Australian Council for Safety and Quality in Health Care (2002) Second national report on patient safety: improving medication safety. AusInfo, Canberra
14. Marzinski P (1991) The tragedy of dementia: clinically assessing pain in the confused, non-verbal elderly. J Gerontol Nurs 17(6):12–19
15. Sengstaken EA, King SA (1993) The problems of pain and its detection among geriatric nursing home residents. J Am Geriatr Soc 41(5):541–544
16. Sindhu F (1996) Are non-pharmacological nursing interventions for the management of pain effective? – a meta-analysis. J Adv Nurs 24:1152–1159
17. McCue JD (1997) Antibiotic resistance: why is it increasing in nursing homes? Geriatrics 52(7):34–36, 39–43
18. Snowdon J, Vaughan R, Miller R, Burgess EE, Tremlett P (1995) Psychotropic drug use in Sydney nursing homes. Med J Aust 163(2):70–72
19. Snowdon J (1998) Management of late-life depression. Australas J Ageing 17(2):57–62
20. Gilbert A, Quintrell LN, Owen N (1988) Use of benzodiazepines among residents of aged-care accommodation. Commun Health Stud 12(4):394–399

21. Robertson MC, Gray JA (1991) Use of benzodiazepines in private nursing homes: a drug 'index' as an indicator of quality in nursing home care. Public Health 105:249–255
22. Ray WA, Taylor JA, Meador KG et al (1993) Reducing antipsychotic drug use in nursing homes: a controlled trial of provided education. Arch Intern Med 153(6):713–721
23. Aronson MK, Cox Post D, Guastadisegni P (1993) Dementia, agitation, and care in the nursing home. J Am Geriatr Soc 41(5):507–512
24. Fonda D (1991) Problems associated with prescribed drug use in the elderly. Aust J Hosp Pharm 21(2):127–130
25. Capezuti E, Talerico KA, Cochran I, Becker H, Strumpf N, Evans L (1999) Individualized interventions to prevent bed-related falls and reduce siderail use. J Gerontol Nurs 25(11): 26–34
26. Leipzig RM, Cumming RG, Tinetti ME (1999) Drugs and falls in older people: a systematic review and meta-analysis: I. Psychotropic drugs. J Am Geriatr Soc 47(1):30–39
27. Avorn J, Soumerai SB, Everitt DE et al (1992) A randomised trial of a program to reduce the use of psychoactive drugs in nursing homes. N Engl J Med 327(3):168–173
28. Gilbert A, Owen N, Innes JM, Sansom L (1993) Trial of an intervention to reduce chronic benzodiazepine use among residents of aged-care accommodation. Aust NZ J Med 23(4):343–347
29. Hunt S (2005) Effective medication management in older people. In: Dunning T (ed) Nursing care of older people with diabetes. Blackwell, Oxford, pp 230–249
30. Lin V (2003) Competing rationalities: evidence-based health policy? In: Lin V, Gibson B (eds) Evidence-based health policy. Oxford University Press, Oxford, pp 3–17
31. Price K (2004) Quality use of medicines [QUM]: are nurses doing what they can and what is it they can do? In: Nursing leadership, policy and politics. Australia National Conference, 14–16 July, 2004, Alice Springs, Northern Territory, Royal College of Nursing, Australia
32. Nichter M, Vuckovic N (1994) Understanding medication in the context of social transformation. In: Etkin NL, Tan ML (eds) Medicines: meanings & context. Health Action Information Network and Medical Anthropology Unit, University of Amsterdam, Netherlands, pp 287–305
33. Hardon AP (1994) Socio-cultural aspects of drug use in the treatment of childhood diarrhea in Oyo State, Nigeria. In: Etkin NL, Tan ML (eds) Medicines: meanings & context. Health Action Information Network and Medical Anthropology Unit, University of Amsterdam, Netherlands, pp 33–46
34. Tan ME, Etkin NL (1994) Introduction. In: Etkin NL, Tan ML (eds) Medicines: meanings & context. Health Action Information Network and Medical Anthropology Unit, University of Amsterdam, Netherlands, pp 1–8
35. Folosade Iyun B (1994) Socio-cultural aspects of drug use in the treatment of childhood diarrhea in Oyo State, Nigeria. In: Etkin NL, Tan ML (eds) Medicines: meanings & contexts. Health Action Information Network and Medical Anthropology Unit, University of Amsterdam, Amsterdam, pp 33–46
36. Sachs L, Tomson G (1994) Brokers, medicines, and rationality: mirroring health centres in Sri Lanka and Sweden. In: Etkin NL, Tan ML (eds) Medicines: meanings & contexts. Health Action Information Network and Medical Anthropology Unit, University of Amsterdam, Amsterdam, pp 263–283
37. World Health Organization (1987) The rational use of drugs. WHO, Geneva
38. World Health Organization (1988) The world drug situation. WHO, Geneva
39. Montague M (1996) The Phamakon phenomenon: cultural conceptions of drugs and drug use. In: Davis P (ed) Contested ground: public purpose and private interested in the regulation of proscription drugs. Oxford University Press, New York, pp 11–25
40. Kawachi I, Conrad P (1996) Medicalization and the pharmacological treatment of blood pressure. In: Davis P (ed) Contested ground: public purpose and private interested in the regulation of prescription drugs. Oxford University Press, New York, pp 26–41
41. Conrad P (1992) Medicalization and social control. Annu Rev Sociol 18:209–232
42. Murray M (1999) What is QUM? In: Hunt S, Parkes R (eds) Nursing and the quality use of medicines. Allen & Unwin, Sydney, pp 1–26

43. Adamson L, Kwok YS, Smith P (1988) Too much of a good thing: older consumers and their medications. Australian Consumers' Association and Combined Pensioners' Association, Melbourne

44. Jones S (1989) Pills, perception and participation – health in older age. Aust J Ageing 8(1):13–17

45. Consumers' Health Forum of Australia (1988) Discussion paper. Rational medicinal drug policy for Australia – what does it mean? Consumers' Health Forum of Australia, Canberra

46. Consumers' Health Forum of Australia (1989) Towards a national medicinal drug policy for Australia. Consumers' Health Forum of Australia, Canberra

47. Roughead E (1998) The suitability of performance indicators for evaluating the implementation and effect of Australia's policy on the quality use of medicines. Unpublished Thesis, University of South Australia, Adelaide, SA

48. Australian Pharmaceutical Advisory Council (1997) Australian Pharmaceutical Advisory Council (APAC) – 1997. Department of Health & Family Services, Canberra

49. Jenkins H (1992) Prescribed health, part 2: prescribing and medication management. House of Representatives Standing Committee on Community Affairs, Australian Government Publishing Service, Canberra

50. Hunt S (2007) Quality use of medicines in residential aged care: an action research study. La Trobe University, Australia

51. Commonwealth Department of Health and Aged Care (1999) National Medicines Policy 2000. http://www.health.gov.au. Accessed 12 Dec 2002

52. Department of Health and Ageing (2002) The national strategy for quality use of medicines. Executive summary. Department of Health and Ageing, Canberra

53. Leeder S (1999) Health medicine: challenges facing Australia's health services. Allen & Unwin, Sydney

54. Consumers' Health Forum of Australia (1999) Understanding consumer behaviour and experiences in relation to the use of medicines. Literature review. Consumers' Health Forum, Canberra

55. Consumers' Health Forum of Australia (2009) Community quality use of medicines project. Seniors and medication safety workshop report. Consumers' Health Forum of Australia, Sydney, Canberra, 12 April 2009

56. Bollen M (2003) Complementary medicines in the Australian health system. Expert committee on complementary medicines in the health system. Report to the Parliamentary Secretary to the Minister for Health and Ageing, Department of Health and Ageing, Canberra

57. Wade T (1999) Consumers or patients – partnerships or compliance? In: Hunt S, Parkes R (eds) Nursing and the quality use of medicines. Allen & Unwin, Sydney, pp 60–72

58. Australian Institute of Health and Welfare (2009) Residential aged care in Australia 2007–2008. A statistical overview. Australian Institute of Health and Welfare, Canberra

59. Goulding MR (2004) Inappropriate medication prescribing for elderly ambulatory care patients. Arch Intern Med 164(2):305–312

60. Australian Pharmaceutical Advisory Council (1997) Integrated best practice model for medication management in residential aged care facilities. Australian Government Publishing Service, Canberra

61. Australian Pharmaceutical Advisory Council (2002) Guidelines for medication management in residential aged care facilities. AusInfo, Canberra

62. Australian Pharmaceutical Advisory Council (2005) Guiding principles to achieve continuity in medication management. AusInfo, Canberra

The Ethics of Prescribing Medications to Older People

David G. Le Couteur, Hal Kendig, Vasi Naganathan, and Andrew J. McLachlan

Keywords Older people • Elderly • Aging • Geriatric pharmacology • Prescribing • Medical ethics • Bioethics • Evidence-based medicine

Medications and Older People

Old age is the major independent risk factor for most diseases of the Western world including atherosclerosis, cancer, and arthritis as well as prototypical aging diseases such as dementia and osteoporosis. Consequently, there is an extensive use of medications among older people who, as a group, are by far and away the greatest consumers of medications in society. Older people use on average 2–5 prescription medications and polypharmacy, defined as the use of five or more medications occurs in 20–40% of this age group [1–4]. While the potential benefits of appropriately prescribed and monitored medications are usually evident [5, 6], there is often limited clinical trial evidence to guide prescribing in the very elderly and frail older person [7, 8]. Furthermore, the hazards and negative outcomes of medications and inappropriate prescribing in older people are well established [6–15]. The incidence of adverse drug reactions correlates with age [16–20] and as many as one-in-five hospital admissions are medication-related in older people [21]. Adverse drug reactions were considered to be the cause of death in about one-in-five older people

---

D.G. Le Couteur (✉)
University of Sydney, Sydney, NSW, Australia
and
Centre for Education and Research on Ageing, Concord
RG Hospital, Concord, NSW, Australia
e-mail: david.lecouteur@sydney.edu.au

S. Koch et al. (eds.), *Medication Management in Older Adults: A Concise Guide for Clinicians*, DOI 10.1007/978-1-60327-457-9_3, © Springer Science+Business Media, LLC 2010

who died while in hospital [22]. Recently, impaired cognitive and physical function in community-dwelling older people were also found to be associated, almost certainly causally, with drug burden [23, 24].

Indubitably, it is of considerable concern that those patients who are prescribed the most medications do not always have a favorable risk to benefit ratio. This paradox has occurred in part because there are inadequate evidence and knowledge about the responses of geriatric patients to medications. Older people are poorly represented in clinical trials with up to 35% of published trials excluding older people on the basis of age without justification [25]. There is an exigent need to increase the number of older and frail people in clinical drug trials and to increase the understanding of the effects of the biological processes of aging on drug action and disposition [13]. Conversely, it has been argued that older people might be denied useful pharmacotherapy because of ageist attitudes and unjustified concerns about adverse effects [26]. Geriatric therapeutics must also take into account specific age-related diseases (dementia, osteoporosis), geriatric syndromes (falls, gait and balance disturbances, incontinence, confusion), and the growing use of antiaging medications. Appropriate prescribing of medications to older people, particularly frail and very elderly patients, is daedal and certainly requires more than unquestioning application of guidelines and systematic reviews designed for younger adults. When confronted with such dilemmas in clinical practice, recourse to medical ethics can provide guidance and subsequent reassurance that any treatment embarked upon is genuinely in the best interest of the patient.

Medical Ethics

Medical ethics encompass the science and philosophy used to identify, analyze, and attempt to resolve moral dilemmas that occur in clinical practice [27, 28]. Among older people, there are distinct ethical issues including those related to competency, resource allocation, therapeutic futility, and end-of-life concerns [27, 29–31]. Many ethical codes have been developed to address such problems dating from the Hippocratic oath and the Prayer of Maimonides to postmodern approaches (e.g., discursive, narrative, feminist, phenomenological philosophies) [29, 32]. All seemingly aim to encapsulate the morality, virtuous and compassionate behavior, and competent decision-making required for the good of the individual and broader community. Over the last few decades, four principles – beneficence, non-maleficence, autonomy, and justice [33, 34] – have come to hold center stage in medical ethics [32]. Although often questioned as the only foundation for medical and bioethics [35, 36], these four principles provide, at minimum, a pragmatic and ecumenical framework to consider ethical problems [32, 34, 35]. Accordingly, these principles can be applied, somewhat simplistically but fruitfully, to the problem of prescribing medications to older people [37, 38].

Beneficence: What Is the Evidence for Efficacy of Medications in Older People?

Beneficence refers to the duty to do good [34]. The principle of beneficence parallels the concept of effectiveness and/or efficacy of medications as defined by evidence-based medicine and clinical trials. From the time of the Hippocrates to the World Medical Association Declaration of Geneva [28], this duty to do good has focused on the individual patient, rather than the broader community. Obviously, there can be overlap and tension between the two. Clinical trials are designed to study groups of patients and correspondingly, any conclusions about treatments refer to the group of subjects with the disease. Guidelines that mandate that all patients with a particular disease must receive a particular treatment are not aligned with the principle of duty of care to the individual patient unless they can guarantee that the recommendation for the group is applicable to the individual. This applies even more to older people, especially frail older people, who are poorly represented in clinical trials in the first place. From the evidence-based medicine perspective, this dilemma is equivalent to the uncertainty about the generalizability of clinical trial results and subsequent individualization of therapies. Even so, in the absence of specific data, advertisements often use pictorial representations of older people presumably to encourage prescribing in this group [39], and some guidelines exhort the greater use of medications in frail older people on the basis of extrapolated benefits [40, 41].

For some medications, the individual prescriber can determine whether good is being done by monitoring the clinical outcome of the patient. Trite examples might include: analgesics for pain, levodopa for Parkinson's disease, diuretics for acute heart failure. However, it is not feasible for a clinician to have any personal experience or insight into whether many, if not most medications, have any efficacy or usefulness [42]. Many medications are designed to reduce the risk of developing illness, and it is almost impossible for a clinician to detect the absence of an illness. Furthermore, the numbers-needed-to-treat for many medications are so large, and the placebo effects are so pervasive that no individual clinician will have prescribed to enough patients to be aware of any impact on outcomes [42] (Table 1). Clinicians are no longer able to rely on their clinical judgment or pharmacological skills to guide their prescribing [42]. Instead, prescribing is guided by information gleaned from clinical trials and provided by journals, guidelines, seminars, marketing, and interactions with colleagues [42].

In the absence of clinical trials performed specifically in geriatric patients and frail older people, subgroup analysis is the next option available to inform the geriatric prescriber. This is justified because there are numerous reasons why geriatric patients might respond differently to medications than typical clinical trial subjects. These reasons include age-related differences in pharmacokinetics, pharmacodynamics, life expectancy, polypharmacy, comorbidity, and disease pathogenesis. There are many problems with subgroup analysis. There is a risk of both false positive and false negative results especially when numerous subgroups are analyzed post hoc.

Table 1 Preventative therapies

Pharmacotherapeutic intervention	Primary outcome	Events over a 12 month period per 100 patients with placebo	Events over a 12 month period per 100 patients with intervention
Antihypertensive therapy [86]	Cardiovascular events and death in older people	3.5	2.5
Bisphosphonates [87]	Vertebral crush fracture	5	3
Bisphosphonates [88]	Hip fracture	0.66	0.33
Angiotensin converting enzyme inhibitors in heart failure [89]	Deaths	13	11
Statins for secondary prevention [90]	Major coronary event	5	4
Aspirin for secondary cardiovascular prevention [91]	Vascular events	13	11
Warfarin in atrial fibrillation [53]	Strokes	4	1.5

The effect of common pharmacotherapeutic interventions on the prevention of clinical outcomes in 100 subjects over 1 year (from [42] with permission). Few, if any clinicians will have enough patients to be able to discern or detect any effect of such medications

If age-interaction analysis is undertaken, then any divergent effect in the oldest cohort can be disguised by the careful selection of the number and size of the other age cohorts. To adequately power a trial to include subgroup analysis, the number of subjects must be substantially increased. With these caveats in mind, it is of interest to examine clinical trials where subgroup analysis has been undertaken to determine whether a differential effect can be discerned in the oldest age groups. Here, older people are defined as more than 75 years of age. Subgroup analyses of subjects aged more than 65 years are probably meaningless for guiding prescribing in geriatric and frail older patients because most contemporary 65- to 75-year-old subjects are considered to be physiologically equivalent to younger adults.

Heart failure medications are an interesting exemplar of the dilemma surrounding evidence, subgroup analysis, and medications in older people [43]. Heart failure is a common condition in older people. About half of people with heart failure are over the age of 75 years, and this group represents nearly 90% of hospital admissions with heart failure. The majority of subjects in heart failure clinical trials are males about 60 years of age with ischemic heart disease and systolic dysfunction. Older people with heart failure are more likely to be females with multifactorial heart disease and diastolic dysfunction. There are also age-related changes in beta-receptors and the renin–angiotensin system that might confound pharmacodynamic responses [13]. Subgroup analyses for the effect of beta-blockers, angiotensin-converting enzyme inhibitors, and eplerenone in heart failure in people over the age of 75 years are shown in Table 2. In all but one case, there was no statistically significant effect on the defined primary outcome in the oldest age groups (in OPTIMIZE-HF, a

Table 2 Results of subgroup analyses for the age group greater than 75 years in heart failure trials

Drug or class	Study	Risk (OR, RR or HR) of primary outcome in subgroup >75 years	Number of subjects >75 years
Angiotensin converting enzyme inhibitors [89]	Meta-analysis of SAVE, AIRE, TRACE and SOLVD	0.89 (0.69–1.13)	1,066
Metoprolol [92]	MERIT-HF	0.79 (0.55–1.14)	490
Nebivolol [93]	SENIORS	0.92 (0.75–1.12)	1,064
Carvedilol [44]	OPTIMIZE-HF observational (combined outcome)	0.79 (0.52–1.20)	939
Carvedilol [44]	OPTIMIZE-HF observational (death)	0.51 (0.29–0.89)	939
Beta-blockers [94]	observational	0.79 (0.52–1.20)	168
Eplerenone [95]	EPHESUS	1.00 (0.75–1.20)	1,326

In all studies, there was a statistically significant effect on the primary outcome for the subgroups less than 75 years of age. The relative risk values for epleronone are approximated from a figure in the US Product Information

nonrandomized observational study, mortality was reduced whereas the combined outcome was not changed) [44]. In all cases, these publications and the reviews and guidelines that have followed, recommend that the medications should be used in all older people with heart failure. The decision as to whether the evidence shows that these medications are effective in heart failure subjects over 75 years hinges on subtleties such as: the value of subgroup analyses; the size and statistical power of the subgroups; the acceptance of confidence intervals crossing unity as a negative result. Application of the ethical principle of beneficence is troublesome because it is not possible to establish from the evidence presented here whether treating an individual patient over 75 years with heart failure does good. Indeed, on first pass, has any efficacy been demonstrated and can beneficence of prescribing these medications really be ensured? To complicate matters even further, a recent review indicated that cardiovascular preventative therapies in older people do not improve life expectancy but merely change the mode of death [45]. Sometimes, this is from a "desirable" death such as sudden death, to a less desirable death by cancer. This reflects the principle of "competing risks" as people get much older. Because old age is the major risk factor for disease, older people have many risk factors for death. Therefore, the absolute effect of reducing the risk of death from one disease has limited effect on overall survival [46].

Another conundrum for the principle of beneficence is polypharmacy. Polypharmacy is usually defined as being present when a patient is taking five or more different medications. There is usually no, or limited evidence supporting the use of multiple medications in the same patient because most clinical trials are performed in uncomplicated patients with single conditions. Even so, there are a few areas where polypharmacy has been shown to be effective, for example, the prevention of cardiovascular disease in people with diabetes mellitus. On the other hand, the adverse effects of polypharmacy have been well described. Of all the age-related factors that increase susceptibility to adverse drug reactions, polypharmacy is considered to be the major factor. The risk of adverse drug reactions increases exponentially with the number of different medications that are taken [8, 13, 47, 48]. Polypharmacy is a risk factor for falls, with those older people taking four or more medications having nearly double the annual risk of falls [47, 48]. Poor adherence and medication administration errors also increase with the number of medications [7, 8, 13]. As an oversimplication, the published evidence shows that polypharmacy can be associated with harm, yet there have been very few trials performed to determine the efficacy of polypharmacy regimens. If clinical trial evidence is the basis for decisions about the good of an intervention and the clinician wishes to apply the principle of beneficence, then polypharmacy should always be avoided.

Nonmaleficence: What Is the Evidence for Harm with Medications in Older People?

Nonmaleficence refers to the duty to prevent or do no harm [33, 34]. For the prescriber, nonmaleficence corresponds with the problem of adverse drug reactions. Similarly, the Hippocratic oath enshrines that "I will neither give a deadly drug to anybody who asked for it, nor will I make a suggestion to this effect." It is unlikely that many clinicians would deliberately prescribe medications to older people in order to cause harm. However, they may do so unknowingly, perhaps influenced by marketing, key opinion leaders, and guidelines that advocate blanket prescribing for specific diseases. Each additional physician who treats an older person increases their risk of an adverse drug reaction by 29% [49]. Adverse drug reactions have been estimated to be between the fourth and sixth leading cause of death in the USA and about half of these deaths were considered to be preventable by better prescribing [50]. Although it is inevitable that any medical intervention will carry some risk, the principle of nonmaleficence demands consideration before any decision is made to prescribe medications, particularly to older people where the risk of adverse drug reactions is increased.

There is evidence that the callow application of the results of clinical trial data to older people can cause harm. What is the real-life outcome when clinical trial data, usually obtained from middle-aged male subjects with a single illness, are applied to frail elderly, often female patients with multiple illnesses? Spironolactone was associated with reduced mortality in clinical trial subjects with heart failure aged about 60 years. When this finding was extrapolated to the general population where most people with heart failure are over 75 years of age, there was an increase in hyperkalemic deaths but no change in heart failure hospitalizations [51]. COX2 inhibitors were associated with reduced risk of gastrointestinal hemorrhages compared to conventional therapies in clinical trial patients, who were mostly younger.

When used in the general population where most people with arthritis are elderly, there was a 10% increase in hospital admissions for gastrointestinal hemorrhage [52]. Warfarin reduces the rate of stroke in clinical trial subjects by about 60% [53], and consequently, the underutilization of warfarin in older people with atrial fibrillation has been extensively criticized [40, 54]. Yet the rate of serious and fatal hemorrhages among nursing home patients on warfarin is so high that the authors of the study concluded that "we believe that the results of this study provide compelling evidence of serious safety concerns around the use of warfarin therapy in the nursing home setting" and calculated that there are 34,000 fatal or serious warfarin-related events among nursing home residents each year in the USA [55]. Similarly, the rate of major hemorrhage in older subjects, commenced on warfarin for atrial fibrillation, was 13% per annum which far exceeds any reduction in absolute stroke rate [56]. The BAFTA study showed overall efficacy of warfarin in older people, yet many of the subjects enrolled in that trial had previously been on warfarin, so there may have been selection bias to include subjects with lower risk of hemorrhage [57]. Spironolactone, anti-inflammatory drugs and warfarin all have type A, predictable, serious adverse drug reactions; yet, they were widely advocated for use in older people despite the biological plausibility of increased adverse reactions in this age group, which was subsequently exposed.

Inappropriate prescribing is a term frequently used in geriatric therapeutics, but admittedly, very difficult to define prospectively [14]. The most commonly cited index of inappropriate prescribing is the Beers criteria, which is a consensus list of medications deemed to be inappropriate when prescribed to older people [58]. The prevalence of inappropriate prescribing as defined by the Beers criteria is high among the elderly, in the range of 10–66% [4, 14, 59–62]. Prescription of inappropriate medications listed by the Beers index to the elderly has been linked in some, but not all, studies to increased rates of adverse drug reactions, death, quality of life, and hospitalization [14] and was even associated with a 31% increase in the risk for nursing home admission [63]. It would appear to be unethical to prescribe medications from the Beers index to older people because there is evidence that these medications cause harm.

There is evidence that polypharmacy is associated with increased risk of adverse drug reactions. For example, in one recent study of 2,018 people over 70 years of age, the odds ratio for adverse drug reactions was 3.4 (95% CI 2.1–5.5) in subjects taking 4–6 medications, 4.6 (95% CI 2.8–7.4) for 7–9 medications, and 5.9 (95% CI 3.6–9.9) for ten or more medications compared with subjects taking 3 or less medications [61]. Polypharmacy is associated with the additive risk of an adverse drug reaction with each successive medication, the increased likelihood of drug interactions [64], and the increased risk of prescribing errors [65]. In a European study, the average number of drugs taken by older people was seven, and 46% had clinically relevant drug interactions, which were considered to be severe in 10% of cases [66]. In a study of 70,203 community dwelling people over 65 years of age taking warfarin, 6.6% were receiving another drug that would be expected to interact with warfarin [67]. Although there are many patient characteristics that predispose to polypharmacy [68], major risk factors include the particular doctor involved in the care of the patient and the total number of doctors who treat the patient [49, 69]. One pathway to polypharmacy is the prescribing cascade where medications are commenced for the management of adverse effects of other medications [70]. Thus, there is an increased risk for starting antihypertensives in subjects on nonsteroidal anti-inflammatory drugs, antigout therapy in subjects taking thiazide diuretics, levodopa in subjects taking metoclopramide [70], and anticholinergic medications in subjects taking cholinesterase inhibitors [71]. Does rational polypharmacy exist or does the evidence indicate that multiple medications are nearly always unethical?

How does one balance nonmaleficence and beneficence, that is, to determine the risk to benefit ratio? In a study of 30,397 person years of community-dwelling older subjects taking medications, the overall rate of adverse drug reactions was 50.1 per 1,000 years. This is equivalent to a number-needed-to-harm of 20 [60]. It would seem rational to avoid any medication in an older person where the evidence for benefit generates a number-needed-to-treat that exceeds 20? In subjects in nursing homes, the rate of adverse drug reactions was even higher at 227 per 1,000 resident years [59]. This yields a number-needed-to-harm of about 4.5, and there are very few medications that generate benefit with a number-needed-to-treat less than this. In other areas of medicine (and evidence-based medicine in general), the focus can be on the efficacy of the medications because adverse drug reactions are less of a concern and certainly less prevalent in younger people. In older people, adverse effects are much more common and severe [8, 23, 59, 60], and therefore it is an ethical duty to consider the principle of nonmaleficence more heedfully before deciding on a therapeutic strategy.

Autonomy: Consent and Older People

Autonomy refers to the duty to respect people and their rights of self-determination [33, 34]. The legal duty to obtain informed consent was developed during court cases in the latter half of the twentieth century where it was decreed that clinicians should provide the information that a reasonable person would need to know in order to make an informed decision about the proposed intervention [27]. To give consent for a treatment, a patient must be able to understand and retain information on the treatment proposed, its indications and its main benefits, as well as possible risk and the consequences of nontreatment, must be shown to believe that information and must be capable of weighing up the information in order to arrive at a conclusion [72].

The issue of informed consent is a particular problem in older people because of the high incidence of dementia. Many patients with dementia are covertly given medications without consent [73, 74]. In a UK study, 71% of residential care facilities and 96% of community carers were prepared to give, or gave medications hidden in food and drink to demented older people, usually without consent or notification of relatives and medical practitioners [72]. Most commonly, this was for psychotropic medications to control behavior, rather than so-called life-saving medications. Obviously, this practice does not comply with the principle of autonomy [73]. Given the increasing recognition of adverse effects of psychotropic drugs in behavioral and psychological symptoms of dementia (stroke, death, diabetes mellitus) [75] and limited if any benefits [76], such administration of psychotropic medications no longer appears to comply with the other principles of beneficence or nonmaleficence.

The issue of competence in dementia is not always an all-or-nothing decision because the degree of cognitive impairment and degree of incompetence can vary with the severity of the illness and intercurrent disease [29]. It is not really possible to estimate what degree of competence is required to make a decision about a particular medication and even so, this would presumably vary according to the risk, benefits, and uncertainties surrounding different medications. And of course, any adjudication of competency (except in extreme cases) is based more on cultural and sociopolitical factors rather than any concrete medical and psychological constructs [77]. One solution is an advanced care directive, but this may have been executed long since and rarely if ever give detailed advice on the use of medications [29]. Anyway, in one randomized study of people with life-threatening illnesses, advance directives had no outcome medical treatments, costs, well being or health status [78].

There are other influences, not necessarily ill intentioned, that impact on treatment decisions by an older person. The term filialism has been coined to describe the limiting of the freedom and autonomy of an older person by well-meaning sons and/or daughters who take over the decision-making process of their parent [30]. However, in many situations, the families wishes regards healthcare and those of the older person are discordant [79]. The momentum and allure of routine medical care and life-extending technologies can also overshadow the choice of an older person to accept or reject a therapeutic option – "the impossibility of saying no to medical interventions" [31]. Of course, the needs of the carer are also taken into consideration when prescribing, particularly with medications given for dementia, psychiatric disorders, and the behavioral and psychological symptoms of dementia. Who makes the decision to treat a person who is deemed incompetent, with a cholinesterase inhibitor or neuroleptic medication? The patient's carer has potentially the most to gain and in fact, the effects of cholinesterase inhibitors on the carer well-being and input time are considered to be appropriate therapeutic outcomes [80]. The patient has potentially the most to lose including possible adverse effects such as death, stroke, incontinence, diabetes mellitus, and myriad gastrointestinal side effects [75, 81]. Yet inevitably, the carer is the surrogate decision-maker, and the patient is considered to be incompetent.

There are manifestly many prescribing situations where the duty to uphold an older persons autonomy and their right to self-determination, is not defended. Although this may occur with the best interests of the patient at heart, ethicists usually concede that autonomy is the chief and most important of the four principles of ethics [32].

Justice: Rationing and the Elderly

Justice refers to the duty to treat individuals fairly, free of bias, and on the basis of medical need [28, 33]. With regard to medications in older people, the obvious issue for the ethical principle of justice relates to allocation of resources [82–84]. It has been argued that medical resources such as medications should be made less available for older people. To support this contention, it is proposed that old people have already lived a full life and it might be unfair to utilize resources to prolong older lives that are already failing, thereby reducing resources for younger people. This is a utilitarian approach to maximize resources for the greatest number of people. However, most younger people who utilize health care resources have serious disease and shortened life expectancy, and, on the other hand, the average life expectancy at 80 years is still another 9 years [82–84]. In addition, the increasing health care costs are largely related to advancing medical technologies rather than increased numbers of sick older people [82]. Although older people may have had a "fair innings" in terms of life expectancy, they have not had access to health care resources that are available and will be available to subsequent cohorts of people [29]. Indeed, because of the association of old age with disease and disability and because older people have had longer to contribute to society, it could easily be asserted that older people should have priority in resource allocation [30, 84]. Regardless of such arguments, the ethical principle of justice ordains that each person's moral claims derive from his or her standing as a human being and are not dependent on any arbitrary factors such as gender, race, or age, and therefore, any age-based allocation of health resources violates the principle of equality [82, 84].

Notwithstanding these ethical principles, the spiraling cost of pharmaceuticals is reducing the ability of older people to access medications. In the USA, a typical older person might have to spend US$9,000 per annum on medications and nearly one in four reporting skipping medications or not filling prescriptions because of this high cost [85]. With regard to the impact of the increasing cost of medications, Marcia Angell wrote "The people hurting the most are the elderly" [85].

Conclusion

The four principles of medical ethics – beneficence, nonmaleficence, autonomy, and justice – provide a pragmatic foundation and steadying influence to guide prescribing in older people where the evidence base for efficacy is uncertain and concerns regarding adverse drug reactions are protean. In most cases, the ethical principles are undermined not by intent, but more likely by lack of knowledge, not only in terms of the knowledge of the individual prescriber, but also the broader evidence and scientific knowledge that underlie geriatric pharmacology. Application of these ethical principles is paramount for those clinicians who publish and promote guidelines and recommendations about prescribing in older people because their capacity to do both good and harm influences the lives and health of many older people.

References

1. Anderson G, Kerluke K (1996) Distribution of prescription drug exposures in the elderly: description and implications. J Clin Epidemiol 49:929–935
2. Jorgensen T, Johansson S, Kennerfalk A, Wallander MA, Svardsudd K (2001) Prescription drug use, diagnoses, and healthcare utilization among the elderly. Ann Pharmacother 35:1004–1009
3. Kennerfalk A, Ruigomez A, Wallander MA, Wilhelmsen L, Johansson S (2002) Geriatric drug therapy and healthcare utilization in the United Kingdom. Ann Pharmacother 36:797–803
4. Shi S, Morike K, Klotz U (2008) The clinical implications of ageing for rational drug therapy. Eur J Clin Pharmacol 64:183–199
5. Ebrahim S (2002) The medicalisation of old age. Br Med J 324:861–863
6. Abernethy DR (1999) Aging effects on drug disposition and effect. Geriatr Nephrol Urol 9:15–19
7. Le Couteur DG, Naganathan V, Cogger VC, Cumming RG, McLean AJ (2006) Pharmacotherapy in the elderly: clinical issues and perspectives. In: Kohli K, Gupta M, Tejwani S (eds) Contemporary perspectives on clinical pharmacotherapeutics. Elsevier, New Delhi, pp 709–722
8. Hilmer SN, McLachlan A, Le Couteur DG (2007) Clinical pharmacology in geriatric patients. Fundam Clin Pharmacol 21:217–230
9. Cumming RG (1998) Epidemiology of medication-related falls and fractures in the elderly. Drugs Aging 12:43–53
10. Walker J, Wynne H (1994) The frequency and severity of adverse drug reactions in elderly people. Age Ageing 23:255–259
11. Denham MJ (1990) Adverse drug reactions. Br Med Bull 46:53–62
12. Mannesse CK, Derkx FH, de Rigger MA, Man in't Veld AJ, van der Cammen TJ (1997) Adverse drug reactions in elderly patients as contributing factor for hospital admissions: cross sectional study. Br Med J 315:1057–1058
13. McLean AJ, Le Couteur DG (2004) Aging biology and geriatric clinical pharmacology. Pharmacol Rev 56:163–184
14. Spinewine A, Schmader KE, Barber N et al (2007) Appropriate prescribing in elderly people: how well can it be measured and optimised? Lancet 370:173–184
15. Routledge PA, O'Mahony MS, Woodhouse KW (2004) Adverse drug reactions in elderly patients. Br J Clin Pharmacol 57:121–126
16. Bordet R, Gautier S, Le Louet H, Dupuis B, Caron J (2001) Analysis of the direct cost of adverse drug reactions in hospitalised patients. Eur J Clin Pharmacol 56:935–941
17. Carbonin P, Pahor M, Bernabei R, Sgadari A (1991) Is age an independent risk factor of adverse drug reactions in hospitalized medical patients? J Am Geriatr Soc 39:1093–1099
18. Hurwitz N (1969) Predisposing factors in adverse reactions to drugs. Br Med J 1:536–539
19. Kellaway GS, McCrae E (1973) Intensive monitoring for adverse drug effects in patients discharged from acute medical wards. N Z Med J 78:525–528
20. Pouyanne P, Haramburu F, Imbs JL, Begaud B (2000) Admissions to hospital caused by adverse drug reactions: cross sectional incidence study. French Pharmacovigilance Centres. Br Med J 320:1036
21. Roughead EE, Gilbert AL, Primrose JG, Sansom LN (1997) Drug-related hospital admissions: a review of Australian studies published 1988-1996. Med J Aust 168:405–408
22. Ebbesen J, Buajordet I, Erikssen J et al (2001) Drug-related deaths in a department of internal medicine. Arch Intern Med 161:2317–2323
23. Hilmer SN, Mager DE, Simonsick EM et al (2007) A drug burden index to define the functional burden of medications in older people. Arch Intern Med 167:781–787
24. Cao YJ, Mager DE, Simonsick EM et al (2008) Physical and cognitive performance and burden of anticholinergics, sedatives, and ACE inhibitors in older women. Clin Pharmacol Ther 83:422–429

25. Bugeja G, Kumar A, Banerjee AK (1997) Exclusion of elderly people from clinical research: a descriptive study of published reports. Br Med J 315:1059
26. (1993) Do doctors short-change people. Lancet 342:1–2
27. Mueller PS, Hook CC, Fleming KC (2004) Ethical issues in geriatrics: a guide for clinicians. Mayo Clin Proc 79:554–562
28. World Medical Association (2005) WMA medical ethics manual. WMA, Ferney-Voltaire
29. Kluge EW (2002) Ethical issues in geriatric medicine: a unique problematic. Health Care Anal 10:379–390
30. Fenech FF (2003) Ethical issues in ageing. Clin Med 3:232–234
31. Kaufman SR, Shim JK, Russ AJ (2004) Revisiting the biomedicalization of aging: clinical trends and ethical challenge. Gerontologist 44:731–738
32. Gillon R (2003) Ethics needs principles – four can encompass the rest – and respect for autonomy should be first among equals. J Med Ethics 29:307–312
33. Beauchamp TL, Childress J (1979) Principles of biomedical ethics, 1st edn. Oxford University Press, New York
34. Gillon R (1994) Medical ethics: four principles plus attention to scope. Br Med J 309:184–187
35. Harris J (2003) In praise of unprincipled ethics. J Med Ethics 23:303–306
36. Campbell AV (2003) The virtues (and vices) of the four principles. J Med Ethics 29:292–296
37. Le Couteur DG, Hilmer SN, Glasgow N, Naganathan V, Cumming RG (2004) Prescribing in older people. Aust Fam Physician 33:777–781
38. Martin FC, O'Mahony MS, Schiff R (2007) Complexity of treatment decisions with older patients: who, when and what to treat? Clin Med 7:505–508
39. Gurnee MC, Hansen JM, Sylvestri MF (1992) Portrayal of the elderly in drug product advertisements: relationship to dosing recommendations and pharmacokinetic data in the geriatric population. J Pharm Mark Manage 7:17–31
40. Adhiyaman V, Kamalakannan D, Oke A, Shah IU, White AD (2000) Underutilization of antithrombotic therapy in atrial fibrillation. J R Soc Med 93:138–140
41. Mangoni AA, Jackson SH (2006) The implications of a growing evidence base for drug use in elderly patients Part 2. ACE inhibitors and angiotensin receptor blockers in heart failure and high cardiovascular risk patients. Br J Clin Pharmacol 61:502–512
42. Le Couteur DG, Kendig H (2008) Pharmaco-epistemology for the prescribing geriatrician. Aust J Ageing 27:3–7
43. Le Couteur DG, Bailey L, Naganathan V (2006) Beta-blockers and heart failure in older people. Eur Heart J 27:887–888
44. Fonarow GC, Abraham WT, Albert NM et al (2007) Carvedilol use at discharge in patients hospitalized for heart failure is associated with improved survival: an analysis from Organized Program to Initiate Lifesaving Treatment in Hospitalized Patients with Heart Failure (OPTIMIZE-HF). Am Heart J 153:82.e1–82.e11
45. Mangin D, Sweeney K, Heath I (2007) Preventive health care in elderly people needs rethinking. BMJ 335:285–287
46. Welch HG, Albertsen PC, Nease RF, Bubolz TA, Wasson JH (1996) Estimating treatment benefits for the elderly: the effect of competing risks. Ann Intern Med 124:577–584
47. Leipzig RM, Cumming RG, Tinetti ME (1999) Drugs and falls in older people: a systematic review and meta-analysis: II. Cardiac and analgesic drugs. J Am Geriatr Soc 47:40–50
48. Leipzig RM, Cumming RG, Tinetti ME (1999) Drugs and falls in older people: a systematic review and meta-analysis: I. Psychotropic drugs. J Am Geriatr Soc 47:30–39
49. Green JL, Hawley JN, Rask KJ (2007) Is the number of prescribing physicians an independent risk factor for adverse drug events in an elderly outpatient population? Am J Geriatr Pharmacother 5:31–39
50. Lazarou J, Pomeranz BH, Corey PN (1998) Incidence of adverse drug reactions in hospitalized patients: a meta-analysis of prospective studies. JAMA 279:1200–1205
51. Juurlink DN, Mamdani MM, Lee DS et al (2004) Rates of hyperkalemia after publication of the Randomized Aldactone Evaluation Study. N Engl J Med 351:543–551

52. Mamdani M, Juurlink DN, Kopp A, Naglie G, Austin PC, Laupacis A (2004) Gastrointestinal bleeding after the introduction of COX 2 inhibitors: ecological study. BMJ 328:1415–1416

53. Aguilar MI, Hart R (2005) Oral anticoagulants for preventing stroke in patients with non-valvular atrial fibrillation and no previous history of stroke or transient ischemic attacks. Cochrane Database Syst Rev CD001927

54. Buckingham TA, Hatala R (2002) Anticoagulants for atrial fibrillation: why is the treatment rate so low? Clin Cardiol 25:447–454

55. Gurwitz JH, Field TS, Radford MJ et al (2007) The safety of warfarin therapy in the nursing home setting. Am J Med 120:539–544

56. Hylek EM, Evans-Molina C, Shea C, Henault LE, Regan S (2007) Major hemorrhage and tolerability of warfarin in the first year of therapy among elderly patients with atrial fibrillation. Circulation 115:2689–2696

57. Mant J, Hobbs FD, Fletcher K et al (2007) Warfarin versus aspirin for stroke prevention in an elderly community population with atrial fibrillation (the Birmingham Atrial Fibrillation Treatment of the Aged Study, BAFTA): a randomised controlled trial. Lancet 370:493–503

58. Fick DM, Cooper JW, Wade WE, Waller JL, Maclean JR, Beers MH (2003) Updating the Beers criteria for potentially inappropriate medication use in older adults: results of a US consensus panel of experts. Arch Intern Med 163:2716–2724

59. Gurwitz JH, Field TS, Avorn J et al (2000) Incidence and preventability of adverse drug events in nursing homes. Am J Med 109:87–94

60. Gurwitz JH, Field TS, Harrold LR et al (2003) Incidence and preventability of adverse drug events among older persons in the ambulatory setting. JAMA 289:1107–1116

61. Laroche ML, Charmes JP, Nouaille Y, Picard N, Merle L (2007) Is inappropriate medication use a major cause of adverse drug reactions in the elderly? Br J Clin Pharmacol 63:177–186

62. Stuart B, Kamal-Bahl S, Briesacher B et al (2003) Trends in the prescription of inappropriate drugs for the elderly between 1995 and 1999. Am J Geriatr Pharmacother 1:61–74

63. Zuckerman IH, Langenberg P, Baumgarten M et al (2006) Inappropriate drug use and risk of transition to nursing homes among community-dwelling older adults. Med Care 44:722–730

64. Mallet L, Spinewine A, Huang A (2007) The challenge of managing drug interactions in elderly people. Lancet 370:185–191

65. Field TS, Mazor KM, Briesacher B, Debellis KR, Gurwitz JH (2007) Adverse drug events resulting from patient errors in older adults. J Am Geriatr Soc 55:271–276

66. Bjorkman IK, Fastbom J, Schmidt IK, Bernsten CB (2002) Drug drug interactions in the elderly. Ann Pharmacother 36:1675–1681

67. Zhan C, Correa-de-Araujo R, Bierman AS et al (2005) Suboptimal prescribing in elderly outpatients: potentially harmful drug-drug and drug-disease combinations. J Am Geriatr Soc 53:262–267

68. Simons LA, Tett S, Simons J et al (1992) Multiple medication use in the elderly. Use of prescription and non-prescription drugs in an Australian community setting. Med J Aust 157:242–246

69. Bjerrum L, Sogaard J, Hallas J, Kragstrup J (1999) Polypharmacy in general practice: differences between practitioners. Br J Gen Pract 49:195–198

70. Rochon PA, Gurwitz JH (1997) Optimising drug treatment for elderly people: the prescribing cascade. Br Med J 315:1096–1099

71. Gill SS, Mamdani M, Naglie G et al (2005) A prescribing cascade involving cholinesterase inhibitors and anticholinergic drugs. Arch Intern Med 165:808–813

72. Treloar A, Beats B, Philpot M (2000) A pill in the sandwich: covert medication in food and drink. J R Soc Med 93:408–411

73. Treloar A, Philpot M, Beats B (2001) Concealing medication in patients' food. Lancet 357:62–64

74. MacDonald AJ, Roberts A, Carpenter L (2004) De facto imprisonment and covert medication use in general nursing homes for older people in South East England. Aging Clin Exp Res 16:326–330

75. Bullock R (2005) Treatment of behavioural and psychiatric symptoms in dementia: implications of recent safety warnings. Curr Med Res Opin 21:1–10

76. Ballard C, Waite J (2006) The effectiveness of atypical antipsychotics for the treatment of aggression and psychosis in Alzheimer's disease. Cochrane Database Syst Rev CD003476

77. Secker B (1999) Labeling patient (in)competence: a feminist analysis of medico-legal discourse. J Soc Philos 30:295–314

78. Schneidermann LJ, Kronick R, Kaplan RM, Anderson JP, Langer RD (1992) Effects of offering advance directives on medical treatments and costs. Ann Intern Med 117:599–606

79. Davis MW, Le Couteur DG, Trim G, Buchanan J, Rubenach S, McLean AJ (1999) Older people in hospital. Aust J Ageing 18(Suppl):26–31

80. Clegg A, Bryant J, Nicholson T et al (2001) Clinical and cost-effectiveness of donepezil, rivastigmine and galantamine for Alzheimer's disease: a rapid and systematic review. Health Technol Assess 5:1–137

81. Kaduszkiewicz H, Zimmermann T, Beck-Bornholdt HP, van den Bussche H (2005) Cholinesterase inhibitors for patients with Alzheimer's disease: systematic review of randomised clinical trials. BMJ 331:321–327

82. Giordano S (2005) Respects for the equality and treatment of the elderly: declarations of human rights and age-based rationing. Camb Q Healthc Ethics 14:83–92

83. Howe EG, Lettieri CJ (1999) Health care rationing in the aged: ethical and clinical perspectives. Drugs Aging 15:37–47

84. Harris J (2005) The age-indifference principle and equality. Camb Q Healthc Ethics 14:93–99

85. Angell M (2005) The truth about drug companies. Scribe, Melbourne

86. Mulrow C, Lau J, Cornell J, Brand M (2000) Pharmacotherapy for hypertension in the elderly. Cochrane Database Syst Rev CD000028

87. Dhesi JK, Allain TJ, Mangoni AA, Jackson SH (2006) The implications of a growing evidence base for drug use in elderly patients. Part 4. Vitamin D and bisphosphonates for fractures and osteoporosis. Br J Clin Pharmacol 61:521–528

88. Nguyen ND, Eisman JA, Nguyen TV (2006) Anti-hip fracture efficacy of biophosphonates: a Bayesian analysis of clinical trials. J Bone Miner Res 21:340–349

89. Flather MD, Yusuf S, Kober L et al (2000) Long-term ACE-inhibitor therapy in patients with heart failure or left-ventricular dysfunction: a systematic overview of data from individual patients. ACE-Inhibitor Myocardial Infarction Collaborative Group. Lancet 355:1575–1581

90. Costa J, Borges M, David C, Vaz Carneiro A (2006) Efficacy of lipid lowering drug treatment for diabetic and non-diabetic patients: meta-analysis of randomised controlled trials. BMJ 332:1115–1124

91. Antithrombotic Triallists Collaboration (2002) Collaborative meta-analysis of randomised trials of antiplatelet therapy for prevention of death, myocardial infarction, and stroke in high risk patients. BMJ 324:71–86

92. Deedwania PC, Gottlieb S, Ghali JK, Waagstein F, Wikstrand JC (2004) Efficacy, safety and tolerability of beta-adrenergic blockade with metoprolol CR/XL in elderly patients with heart failure. Eur Heart J 25:1300–1309

93. Flather MD, Shibata MC, Coats AJ et al (2005) Randomized trial to determine the effect of nebivolol on mortality and cardiovascular hospital admission in elderly patients with heart failure (SENIORS). Eur Heart J 26:215–225

94. Dobre D, DeJongste MJ, Lucas C et al (2007) Effectiveness of beta-blocker therapy in daily practice patients with advanced chronic heart failure; is there an effect-modification by age? Br J Clin Pharmacol 63:356–364

95. US product information for Inspra. Accessed at http://www.pfizer.com/files/products/uspi_inspra.pdf

Common Medication Errors in the Acute Care Sector

Susan Koch, Helen Forbes, and Pauline Wong

Keywords Medication errors • Older people • Acute care • Medication management

Human Interaction Issues That May Lead to Errors and Strategies to Overcome

Complexity causes errors. Researchers who have studied this relationship have developed operational definitions of complexity of a task using measures that include steps in the task, number of choices, duration of execution, information content and patterns of intervening, distracting tasks. These measures provide a convenient list of factors to consider when simplifying individual tasks or multi-task processes [1–4].

It is recognized that errors in medication prescription, dispensing and administration occur because of multiple factors rather than any single cause [5]. Adverse events or errors occur when there is a combination of "active failures" and "latent conditions." Reason [6] defines active failures as "slips, lapses, fumbles, mistakes and procedural violations." Latent conditions, according to Reason, occur within the system as a consequence of management decisions or building and design problems, among others. The interaction of active failures and latent conditions contributes to the occurrence of errors [7–9]. The effect of high workloads, fatigue, staff stress, poor communication, inexperience and poorly maintained or inadequate equipment in combination with "active failures" predisposes to errors. Not all medication management errors result in harm. Errors that do result in injury are sometimes called preventable adverse events. Errors that do not result in harm also

S. Koch (✉)
Australian Centre for Evidence Based Aged Care, c/ Bundoora Extended Care Centre,
1231 Plenty Road, Bundoora, Victoria 3083, Australia
e-mail: s.koch@latrobe.edu.au

S. Koch et al. (eds.), *Medication Management in Older Adults:*
A Concise Guide for Clinicians, DOI 10.1007/978-1-60327-457-9_4,
© Springer Science+Business Media, LLC 2010

represent an important opportunity to identify system improvements having the potential to prevent adverse events. Preventing medication errors means designing medication management policies, guidelines and protocols at all points of the management process to make it safer.

Environmental Interaction Issues That May Lead to Errors and Strategies to Overcome

The environment in which medications are prescribed, prepared, stored and administered is just as critical to patient safety as is the suitability and appropriateness of the medication for the particular patient, the person who prescribes the medication and the person who administers the medication. Of importance also is the fact that acute care clinical settings are becoming increasingly complex environments. Anderson and Webster [7] report that errors with the administration of medications are partly due to the increase in type and number of available drugs and different methods of administration in particular. An example of this is evident with the variety of routes, which can be used to administer analgesia. These routes include topical, oral, subcutaneous, intramuscular, intravenous (IV), intrathecal and rectal. The route selected requires specific knowledge and skill about drug actions, effect on patient, technique used and so on. To further guide the health care professional in relation to selecting the most appropriate route of drug administration, knowledge about the impact of normal aging and pathological changes on pharmacokinetics and pharmacodynamics is essential. The cognitive ability of the patient is another important factor when deciding upon the most appropriate route for administration of medication. For example, for someone experiencing a delirium, IV medication may not be the most appropriate route because it may increase the level of agitation and distress being experienced.

Some specific features of the clinical work environment have been identified as contributing to medication errors. For example, environmental contributors include the inadequate labelling of drugs [7, 9], drug cupboard/trolleys that are cluttered and overstocked, incomplete prescriptions [7, 10]. Illegible prescriptions, medication charts and charts waiting to be rewritten were also identified as contributing to errors [9, 10]. Leape [11] provides some examples of a complexity inducing resulting from personal preference. These include non-therapeutic differences in drug doses and times of administration, different locations for stored medications and different equipment on different units.

The impact of the environment is an important consideration for minimizing medication errors in acute care settings. The medication process depends on systems being in place to ensure the patient is appropriately and safely treated [12]. Even though administration of medications is often planned, distractions and interruptions can be enough for an error to occur. Interruptions from patients or colleagues or having to answer the telephone are specific examples provided by Fry and Dacey [10]. The likelihood of error is further increased if the staff member is fatigued, inexperienced and/or has a high patient load [9]. The combination of individual health care team members, the patient and the person who prescribes, dispenses, stores or administers medication and the clinical work environment provides opportunities for errors to occur. Consideration should also be given in units where there are patients experiencing unmet needs behaviours (challenging behaviours) causing disruptions during administration. Although not identified as best practice, a management strategy could be allocation of additional staff at times of high drug administration.

A common approach to the management of medication errors has been to focus on individuals by singling out and disciplining those deemed to be responsible [6]. A major shift of focus must take place, where, instead of blaming individuals for past medication errors to focus on preventing future medication errors by designing safety into the system. This does not mean that individuals can be careless. People must still be vigilant and held responsible for their actions. But when an error occurs, blaming an individual does little to make the system safer and prevent someone else from committing the same error. To err is human, but errors can be prevented.

Anderson and Webster [7] recommend a quality program of continuous improvement where aspects of the clinical environment are redesigned and monitored to facilitate safe and efficient administration of medications. To redesign features of the clinical drug prescription, storage and administration environment, it is important to investigate where the weaknesses are in this aspect of the system. Investigations are more likely to reveal weakness in the system where there is a culture of ongoing reporting and feedback. Such an approach places responsibility for safety on all members of the health care team responsible for handling medications. In such a culture, it is necessary to learn from mistakes. A culture of safety is where the staff work in teams providing an environment where questions about medication practices and processes can be raised [12]. Reason [6] strongly urges organizations to expect errors as they are part of human nature. In recognition of this, it is recommended that each organization establishes a level of performance in relation to errors and adverse events. Nolan [13] recommends that an aim should be to have no instances of errors causing harm to patients. He further identifies the need to design the system to prevent errors from occurring, make errors more visible so that action can be taken to prevent harm to the patient and lessen the effect of errors when they occur but are not detected. To achieve such an outcome, the focus is shifted from blaming the individual to training staff to recognize errors and to look at ways in which the system has failed.

Designers of systems of care can make them safer by attending to three tasks: designing the system to prevent errors, designing procedures to make errors visible when they do occur so that they may be intercepted and designing procedures for mitigating the adverse effects of errors when they are not detected and intercepted [14–18].

Inspection or "double checking" such as the inspection of medication orders (prescriptions) by the pharmacist and the checking of a nurse's dose calculations by another nurse or by a computer are examples of making errors visible. If patients are educated about the course of their treatment and their medications in the context of a trusting relationship, patients can also be effective at identifying errors. They should be encouraged to ask questions and to speak up when unusual circumstances arise.

Not all errors will be intercepted before reaching the patient. When errors go undetected, processes are needed that quickly reverse or halt the harm caused to the patient. For example, antidotes for high hazard drugs, when they exist, should be readily available at the point of administration. Lessons learnt from other more frequently used emergency procedures, such as resuscitation of a patient in cardiac arrest, will be helpful to develop these procedures.

Technical Interaction Issues That May Lead to Errors and Strategies to Overcome

Storage and administration of medications in the acute care sector is commonly associated with the use of technologies such as IV infusion pumps, including new generation "smart" pumps, automatic dispensing cabinets/devices and robotic dispensing technology. Hospitals are also now investing in complex integrated clinical information and medication management systems, that may include bar code scanning devices, computerized physician order entry (CPOE) systems and personal digital assistants to monitor and control any one or more of the processes involved in prescribing, dispensing, storing or administering medications.

One of the underlying rationales for using technologies to support medication practices is to reduce the risk of adverse events, particularly those related to human error such as administering the wrong drug, the wrong dose or administering a drug to the wrong patient. However, despite the increasing uptake of such technologies in the acute care sector, medication errors continue to occur and there is poor evidence to support that technologies used to store and administer medications do in fact reduce the risk of medication errors [19, 20].

Medications delivered via the IV route have been found to present the greatest potential for harm. This is not surprising considering the fast onset of action and potential for serious side effects associated with these drugs [21, 22]. In addition, critically ill patients and those receiving IV infusions or "high alert" medications (e.g. heparin, insulin, dopamine, propofol, antineoplastics) are at an increased risk of life-threatening consequences to adverse drug events [23, 24]. Older people require increased vigilance due to the increased number of medications prescribed, alterations in metabolism with age and the existence of other medical problems and comorbidities [25]. The potential for serious harm or even death as a consequence of medication errors in these populations and involving these drugs cannot be underestimated.

Sources of error related to storage and administration of IV drug infusions include preparation of the wrong infusion concentration or the use of the wrong diluents, storage of potentially lethal drugs in the patient's bedside drawers (e.g. IV potassium chloride) and the transfer of patients between departments with poorly labelled drug infusions [26]. For example, critically ill patients may have up to a dozen IV infusion lines. The risk of an adverse drug event is increased when patients are transferred from the ICU to the operating theatre without clearly identifying each line. Similarly, when departments within a hospital have different drug infusion concentration protocols and methods of delivery, the potential for error may be increased during interdepartmental patient transfers.

Taxis [22] explored causes of IV medication errors and found that 73% of errors occurred when giving bolus doses and that nurses intentionally injected drugs faster than recommended guidelines. Causes cited included a lack of perceived risk, poor role models and available technology. Other mistakes occurred when drug administration or preparation involved uncommon procedures such as the preparation of small volumes or unusual drug vial preparations. The lack of knowledge related to preparation or administration and complex design of equipment were considered sources for these mistakes. For example, misreading the drug label or if two separate vials were provided to prepare the one dose.

Standard IV infusion pumps are commonly used in the acute care setting to prevent errors associated with administering medications via the IV, epidural and subcutaneous routes. Medications administered via these routes can include narcotic analgesics for pain relief, local and general anesthetics during surgery and inotropes to provide haemodynamic support to the critically ill patient in shock. Administration of medications and fluids via an IV infusion pump is intended to deliver an accurate dose of the drug or fluid at the correct rate.

Medication errors related to the use of standard IV infusion pumps include the lack of knowledge related to the functionality, set-up or adjustment of the infusion device [21–23, 27]. Poor practical skills and knowledge related to IV pump use may lead to the incorrect dose or accidental bolus doses being administered [23]. The design of the pump, such as the front panel user interface, can cause confusion particularly when there are multiple channels within the one device or if the channels are not labelled clearly [26].

"Smart pumps" have been designed to reduce the potential for serious adverse events related to programming errors associated with standard IV pumps. These advanced infusion therapy systems incorporate institution-defined medication lists and standard concentrations that are pre-programmed into the machine. Safety software that recognize preset "hard" limits that cannot be overridden and "soft" limits that may be overridden at the clinician's discretion, as well as minimum and maximum dosages, provide alerts that warn or prevent the clinician from inadvertently programming an incorrect dose, rate or volume of drug. However, like any technology, their potential for improving medication safety can only be realized if the clinicians use the technology appropriately, question suggestions made by the computer and decisions continue to be informed by clinical expertise.

Rothschild et al. [20] performed a prospective, randomized time-series trial comparing the serious medication error rate between IV pumps with active decision support software to a control group with decision support turned off. No reduction in the rate of serious medication errors was found. The authors believed this was due to pump design and clinical practices that bypassed the safety features of the pumps. For example, overriding the drug library knowledge base preventing the pumps from checking limits or providing feedback warnings.

To prevent such medication errors associated with technology, it is imperative that human factors are considered in the design and development of such products. The user interface should be as simple as possible to minimize the number of steps required to set an infusion rate or to deliver a bolus. Similarly, features that prevent clinicians from taking short cuts and overriding the safety features should be considered. In the above example, the design of the pump was such that the drug library inactivated was the default setting when the pump was initially set up. Changing the default to have the drug library activated reduced the chance of nurses overriding this feature from the start [20].

A major cause of medication errors is lack of information about the patient that can lead to poor decision making with regard to medication prescribing and administration. For example, information such as laboratory results, the patient's weight, allergies, comorbidities and other data may be needed to make decisions about dose prescription or patient tolerance to a particular drug.

Comprehensive medication management systems may include bar code-enabled medication administration (BCMA), electronic medication administration records (e-MAR) and CPOE systems that interface with other patient information systems such as laboratory results or an electronic health record (EHR). These systems can provide vital, "real time" information for both the physician prescribing and the nurses administering the medication to prevent medication errors in the acute care setting [28]. A "bar code system... coupled with a computerized order entry system would greatly enhance the ability of all health care workers to follow the 'five rights'" [29]. A patient's bar coded wristband would contain information about the patient's treatment plan, medical history, drug allergies and medication administration record. The nurse, using a hand-held scanning device would scan the bar code on the drug, the patient's ID wristband and the nurse's own ID badge. The scanning device connected via a wireless network to a mainframe computer would update the patient's treatment plan and medication record accordingly. As a result, the right patient would receive the right drug and dose at the right time and via the right route, and documentation would be up to date and accurate at all times [29].

Automatic Dispensing Cabinets (ADCs) are widely used throughout the Emergency Department (ED) in the USA. They have been introduced to improve pharmacy inventory, billing, distribution and dispensing processes and to increase the security of narcotics. Vendors suggest that ADCs also reduce drug costs and improve efficiency and patient safety. However, despite their purported benefits, medication errors associated with the use of ADCs continue to occur.

Potential sources of error associated with the use of ADCs include:

- Overstocking with an excessive number of vials or dose strengths of a particular drug enabling greater strengths of a drug to be prepared by mistake. The chance of unused medications expiring more readily is also increased.
- The storage of adult and paediatric forms of medication in the same ADC or when the wrong drug is mixed up in the matrix drawer of another drug.
- The ability of clinicians to remove drugs from the cabinet without consulting the patient's medication record.
- Elimination of the usual "gatekeeping" function of the pharmacist, who uses pharmacy computer systems to cross-check the prescription with the patient's weight, allergies, comorbidities and drug interactions [19, 30].

Strategies to overcome errors associated with the use of ADCs include ensuring an adequate number of ADCs are provided and strategically placed around the ED. This prevents nurses from taking several drugs for multiple patients at once to avoid walking down long corridors. In addition, if the ED services a large paediatric population, separate ADCs stocked with paediatric doses should be provided for those patients. The use of bar coding technology, as mentioned previously, integrated with the ADC can assist in the stocking, retrieval and administration processes. Minimizing the variety of drug concentrations, avoiding bulk supplies, stocking with ready to use, clearly labelled unit doses and restocking more frequently will also reduce the risk of error. Only trained pharmacy staff should be permitted to restock the cabinets and double checking of "high alert" medications should be enforced [19].

Conclusion

It is widely accepted that the use of new technologies in the acute care sector will improve patient safety and reduce the risk of medication errors [31]. However, despite their promise of being a panacea for medication safety issues, many of these technologies may potentially provide an alternative source for medication errors, and the real benefits for the patient will only be recognized if clinicians are educated in their proper use, the technology is appropriately applied and human factors are considered in their design and evaluation.

While medication management systems may overcome many problems related to prescribing, dispensing and administration of medications, availability is inconsistent. In environments where such systems are not available, some practical strategies are provided in Table 1, which may reduce the likelihood of medication errors.

Table 1 Interaction breakdown that causes medication management errors during prescribing, dispensing, administration and storage and strategies to support a reduction in medication management errors

Error	Active failure/error producing conditions	Best practice principles
Prescribing	Illegible handwriting	Write clearly: *print it*
Dispensing	Memory lapse	Fill in *all* the boxes that you are required to on the chart
Administration	Fatigue	
Storage	Inadequately trained staff	Use a *reliable* data source: do not rely on your memory; calculate, do not estimate; check interactions
	Use of non-standard abbreviations in drug prescriptions [13]	
		Remember to modify the dosage for the older person
	Non-conducive environment	
	(In environments such as *or* where verbal orders are issued)	Use *accepted* abbreviations: dose, frequency, timing, route,: units of measure and concentration and dose format
	Lapses in following policy and evidence-based clinical guidelines	Keep chart numbers to a *minimum*
		Listen when someone raises concerns
	Incorrect identity checking	*Record* on a whiteboard (mounted and visible to all staff)
	Medications that look the same	*Read* the order back to the prescriber for approval
	Medications that sound the same	*Purposeful space*: well lit; no through traffic
	Medications that are highly dangerous	*Concentrate*: ENFORCE no interruptions and focus on medication prescribing
		Minimize interruptions:
		Other staff respect the importance of the task you are undertaking
		Where possible *double check* medications being administered
		Refer to organizational policies; safety reminders and checklists
		Provide quiet workplaces for preparation of medications [13] and adequate lighting [12]
		Use of medication administration technologies, e.g. bar code-enabled medication administration to ensure the patient receives the medication according to the "five rights" [32]
		Use of *colour coding* to differentiate between size and shape of similar medications [13]
		Elimination of drugs that have similar sounding names [13]
		Remove concentrated electrolytes, i.e. potassium from clinical areas [13]

References

1. Wichman H, Oyasato A (1983) Effects of locus of control and task complexity on prospective remembering. Hum Factors 25:583–591 (Medline)
2. Maylor EA, Rabbitt GH, James GH, Kerr SA (1992) Effects of alcohol, practice, and task complexity on reaction time distributions. Q J Exp Psychol 44A:119–139
3. Hinckley CM, Barkman P (1995) The role of variation, mistakes, and complexity in producing nonconformities. J Qual Technol 27:242–249
4. Fraass B, Lash K, Matrone G, Volkman SK, McShan DL, Kessler ML et al (1998) The impact of treatment complexity and computer-control delivery technology on treatment delivery errors. Int J Radiat Oncol Biol Phys 42:651–659 (Medline)
5. Fry M, Dacey C (2007) Factors contributing to incidents in medicine administration. Part 1. Br J Nurs 16(9):556–559
6. Reason J (2000) Human error: models and management. Br Med J 320:768–770
7. Anderson DJ, Webster CS (2001) A systems approach to the reduction of medication error on the hospital ward. J Adv Nurs 35(1):34–41
8. Vincent C (2003) Understanding and responding to adverse events. N Engl J Med 348(11):1051–1056
9. Mayo A, Duncan D (2004) Nurse perceptions of medication errors: what we need to know for patient safety. J Nurs Care Qual 19(3):209–217
10. Fry M, Dacey C (2007) Factors contributing to incidents in medicine administration. Part 2. Br J Nurs 16(11):676–681
11. Leape L (1994) Error in medicine. JAMA 272:1851–1857 (CrossRef) (Medline)
12. McBride-Henry K, Foureur M (2007) A secondary care nursing perspective on medication administration safety. J Adv Nurs 60(1):58–66
13. Nolan T (2000) System changes to improve patient safety. Br Med J 320:771–773
14. Salvendy G (1997) Handbook of human factors and ergonomics. Wiley, New York
15. Norman DA (1988) The psychology of everyday things. Basic Books, New York
16. Norman DA (1993) Things that make us smart. Addison-Wesley, New York
17. Leveson NG (1993) Safeware, systems safety and computers. Addison-Wesley, New York
18. Leape L, Bates D, Cullen D, Cooper J, Demonaco HJ, Gallivan T et al (1995) Systems analysis of adverse drug events. JAMA 274:35–43 (Abstract)
19. Paparella S (2006) Automated medication dispensing systems: not error free. J Emerg Med 32(1):71–74
20. Rothschild JM, Keohane CA et al (2005) A controlled trial of smart infusion pumps to improve medication safety in critically ill patients. Crit Care Med 33(3):533–540
21. Kremsdorf R (2003) Using innovation technology to enhance patient care delivery. Nurs Outlook 51(3):S16–S20
22. Taxis K, Barber N (2003) Causes of intravenous medication errors: an ethnographic study. Qual Saf Health Care 12:343–348
23. Brush K (2003) Upgrading systems design to reduce medication administration errors. Clin Nurse Spec 17(1):15–16
24. Dennison RD (2007) A medication safety education program to reduce the risk of harm caused by medication errors. J Contin Educ Nurs 38(4):176–184
25. Hughes RG, Ortiz E (2005) Medication errors: why they happen, and how they can be prevented. Am J Nurs 105:14–24
26. Burdeau G, Crawford R, Van de Vreede M, McCann J (2006) Taking aim at infusion confusion. J Nurs Care Qual 21(2):151–159
27. Ulumino VM, O'Leary-Kelly C, Connolly P (2007) Nurses perception of causes of medication errors and barriers to reporting. J Nurs Care Qual 22(1):28–33
28. Mullen J (2005) Technology as an aid to the nurse–patient interaction at the bedside. Am J Nurs 39:1–6

29. Roark DC (2004) Bar codes and drug administration: can new technology reduce the number of medication errors? Am J Nurs 104(1):63–66
30. Wolf ZR (2007) Pursuing safe medication use and the promise of technology. MedSurg Nurs 16(2):92–100
31. Crane J, Crane FG (2006) Preventing medication errors in hospitals through a systems approach and technological innovation: a prescription for 2010. Res Perspect Healthcare 84(4):3–8
32. Englebright JD, Franklin M (2005) Managing a new medication administration process. J Nurs Adm 35(9):410–413

Common Medication Errors in Long-Term Care Settings

Catherine Edgar and Penny Harvey

Keywords Long-term care setting • Residential aged care facility • Aged care home • Nursing home • Skilled nursing facility • Medication management • Medication error • Medication and older people

Medication Errors and Their Impact

There are numerous definitions offered for what constitutes a medication error and there is a wide variation in the rates of medication error reported in studies of medication preparation and administration in hospitals which can be explained by the differences in definitions used to describe a medication error [1, 2]. Furthermore, the term "adverse drug reaction" or "adverse effect" is often used interchangeably in the literature and depending on how researchers report their findings, can be confusing and at times appear to be contradictory in its use [3, 4]. An adverse drug reaction has been defined by the World Health Organisation [5] as: "Any response to a drug which is noxious, unintended and occurs at doses used for prophylaxis, diagnosis or therapy".

For clarity, a medication error is "any preventable event that may cause or lead to inappropriate medication use or patient harm while the medication is in the control of a health professional, patient or consumer" [3].

It is estimated that in Australia in 2007, approximately 180,000 people experienced an adverse effect from medicines that required hospitalisation. While in the hospital, another 2% of patients experience harm or die as a result of medication errors [6]. It has been suggested that medication errors (mistakes or lapses when medications are prescribed, dispensed or used) are by and large potentially preventable [7]. Medication errors pose serious implications for all health personnel involved in the prescribing, dispensing and administration of medications as the

C. Edgar (✉)
Bundoora Extended Care Centre, 1231 Plenty Road, Bundoora, Victoria 3083, Australia
e-mail: Catherine.edgar@nh.org.au

S. Koch et al. (eds.), *Medication Management in Older Adults: A Concise Guide for Clinicians*, DOI 10.1007/978-1-60327-457-9_5, © Springer Science+Business Media, LLC 2010

risk for medication errors is increasing with the use of more complex drug regimens and potent medications associated with the increasing age and co-morbidities of patients [8, 9].

Age-related physiological changes such as altered pharmacodynamics and pharmacokinetics can impact on an older person's ability to clear and excrete drugs from the body [10]. This increases the potential for adverse effects of medications. Also, because older people generally have multiple co-morbidities, they are more likely to be taking a variety of medications; once a person takes four or more regular medications, the potential for adverse effects increases exponentially [11, 12]. Several other papers have reported a similarly strong correlation between higher numbers of medications per person and the rates of adverse drug reactions [13–16]. In most cases, the adverse effects of medications are unpredictable and those that do occur can be explained by a drug–drug interaction, by the cumulative side effects of a drug that alone would not cause significant morbidity and, to some extent, by an increased risk of medication error [3].

Each year, approximately 30% of people aged 75 years and older are admitted to hospitals with medication-related issues that may range from minor discomfort to a major life-threatening event [10, 12, 17]. However, even minor discrepancies in the administration of medication to older people can have very serious and negative outcomes [18]. Older people living in long-term care facilities take more prescription medications than their peers living in the community. This places them at an even higher risk of experiencing an adverse drug reaction and medication error with the potential for worse outcomes [19–23].

Medication management in long-term care settings is a complex process confounded by the very nature of the setting itself. There is evidence to suggest that at each step along the continuum from prescription to medication delivery to the resident, there is the potential for substantial errors to be made that may result in serious consequences for the resident concerned. Although the issues surrounding medication management and factors that contribute to medication errors in hospital settings have been extensively researched, there are relatively few studies that focus on medication errors in long-term care settings.

Long-term care facilities are generally purpose-built residential facilities that cater to the needs of older people in terms of providing personal care and other support services such as pharmacy, allied health or specialist services. In Australia, there are two designated levels of care provided in long-term care facilities; "low care" and "high care". Residents who require some assistance with the activities of everyday living such as, hygiene, grooming and general housekeeping tasks receive low care. Whereas residents whose personal care needs are greater and who may require specialised nursing care to ensure their needs are met receive high care [24]. All residents, regardless of level of care are offered assistance and supervision with medication management including supply, packaging and administration.

Long-term care facilities are required to employ an adequate number of staff with an appropriate mix of skills and qualifications to ensure that residents receive the care that they need. However, staffing ratios and skill mix in long-term care facilities are significantly different to the hospital setting with a great variation in skill mix across facilities. The staffing and skill mix depends on the particular facility and the level of care provided; staffing profiles can include a mixture of Division 1 Registered Nurses (Div 1 RNs), Enrolled Nurses (Div 2 RNs), or Patient Care Assistants (PCAs). Long-term care facilities providing a high level of care are required to have a Div 1 RN on duty at all times to co-ordinate, supervise and manage the administration of medication to residents. Whereas, in long-term care facilities that provide low level care, the administration of medications to residents may be the sole responsibility of a PCA, with associated restrictions on the formulations and routes of medications that can be administered [25].

What causes medication errors to occur has been extensively studied with most studies reporting that there are multiple contributing factors implicated in the development of medication errors and that there is no one single strategy that will successfully prevent their occurrence in all situations [26–28]. Although most studies related to medication errors have been conducted in the hospital or community setting, most study findings could be generalised to long-term care settings as the contributing factors identified in the hospital setting are similar and equally applicable to long-term care settings.

There are, however, some very important differences between hospitals and long-term care facilities that make the overall management of medication in long-term care settings precarious. Most long-term care facilities lack the same supportive infrastructure as the hospital setting. In addition to differences in staffing ratios and skill mix, access to pharmaceutical, medical and pathology services are limited compared to the typical hospital setting, as all of these services are off-site. This makes the long-term care setting a potentially more hazardous, high-risk environment with an increased potential for serious medication errors to occur anywhere along the continuum, from prescription of medications to administration of medication to a resident.

Causes of Medication Errors

There are recurring themes in the literature on the subject of the causes and contributing factors related to the incidence of medication errors. There is a general consensus that a breakdown in or lack of systems and processes that ensure medication is managed safely is a significant contributing factor involved in medication errors. Other causes that have been cited relate to errors in all stages of the medication process: errors in the prescription of medication, errors in the supply of medications and errors in the administration of medications, including a variety of human factors [28–32].

While nurses have identified human error and poor communication as a significant cause of medication errors, they are seldom the result of one person's actions alone [33]. Medication errors are often the result of multiple breakdowns in the systems or processes in place. When a root cause analysis of a medication error has been conducted, the origin and contributing factors that resulted in that error are often revealed to be multifactorial and involve a mixture of human error with deficiencies in systems and processes [26, 34]. Chassin and Becher [20] analysed a case where a patient mistakenly underwent an invasive test, which included the administration of medication. In their analysis, they discovered at least 17 distinct errors that contributed to the "wrong patient" scenario; this highlights how no one single error caused the mistake in itself.

Types of Errors

Prescribing errors in medication are found across all settings; community, hospital and long-term care facilities. The most commonly identified medication errors in prescribing relate to the prescription of inappropriate drugs, errors in calculating dosage, infrequent monitoring of the therapeutic effects of medication, errors in the duplication of medications relating to the use of brand name drugs versus generic name drugs and errors related to illegible drug orders [2, 28, 35, 36].

Errors in Prescription

Prescribing medications to older patients requires special consideration because of the associated aged related physiological changes and often, multiple co-morbidities. While many prescription drugs have considerable potential to reduce morbidity and mortality and improve functioning in older people, careful consideration must be given to the dose prescribed as the potential for an untoward adverse effect increases with ageing [37].

Older people in long-term care facilities are twice as likely to receive inappropriate prescriptions compared to their peers living in the community, and it has been estimated that between 16 and 50% of older people in long-term care settings receive one or more inappropriate prescriptions annually [4, 38]. While it may be unrealistic to expect any physician to be conversant with all the tens of thousands of prescriptions and over-the-counter medications on the market [39], making use of the Beers criteria when prescribing medications for older people would help alert and prompt doctors to consider the appropriateness of the medications they prescribe.

The Beers criteria are a consensus-based list of medications identified as potentially inappropriate for use in older adults. The criteria were introduced in 1991 to help researchers evaluate prescription quality in nursing homes [40, 41]. Unless doctors are familiar with the Beers criteria, there is a strong possibility that some medications prescribed to older people in long-term care could be considered inappropriate and increase the potential for an adverse drug reaction to occur. The Beers criteria is discussed further in the Chapter "Inappropriate Prescribing: Beers Criteria, Polypharmacy, and Drug Burden".

A study by Gurwitz et al. [10] revealed that most medication errors were associated with prescription and drug monitoring. The most common errors related to the wrong dose followed by the wrong choice of drug and known drug interactions. Almost half of the events were classified as fatal, life threatening or serious. Other studies support this finding and have shown that medication errors usually occur during the prescription and administration stages. More than 80% of adverse drug reactions precipitating or occurring during hospital admissions are dose-related in nature and are therefore potentially avoidable [37, 42, 43].

Look Alike, Sound Alike Medications

Look alike, sound alike medications are common causes of medication errors, and there is a strong likelihood that the wrong medication may be administered because of the similarities of some drug names and packaging. For example, medications with similar names like Oxynorm (oxycodone) instead of Oxazepam, or Gliclizide instead of Glipizide, Losec (omeprazole) and Lasix (furosemide) are problematic worldwide. To reduce confusion and the potential for a medication error to occur, policies need to be in place that requires the treating doctor to use both the non-proprietary name and the brand name of the medication when prescribing [44].

Illegible Drug Orders

Illegible or ambiguous medication orders are often cited as a cause of medication errors and nurses frequently report their dissatisfaction with poorly written and illegible prescriptions [45]. It is the responsibility of nurses to consult with the doctor who prescribes the medication to clarify the order and request that the drug name and dose be printed clearly prior to administering the medication to the resident to ensure it is administered safely and in accordance with best practice and professional codes of conduct. One strategy that has been used successfully to reduce errors related to illegible medication orders is the implementation of an electronic medication ordering system. The introduction of an electronic medication ordering system in four long-term care facilities has been shown to reduce or eliminate errors related to illegible handwriting [46]. An electronic medication ordering system also has the capacity to provide doctors with an automated prompt regarding possible adverse drug interactions [47].

Infrequent Monitoring

An essential part of medication management is to monitor the therapeutic effects of medication, particularly in older people who are more vulnerable to the potential toxic effects of medications [1, 48]. For example, insulin, warfarin, antibiotics and diuretics are medications that are commonly prescribed to older people and are considered high-risk medications [49]. High-risk medications have narrow therapeutic indices or small margins of safety and require close and regular monitoring to ensure that medication doses are within acceptable therapeutic ranges [50, 51]. Other medications that require close monitoring include anticonvulsants, antipsychotics, benzodiazepines and opiate analgesics. It is recommended that every resident should have a regular (at least annually) comprehensive medication review conducted in collaboration with a pharmacist, the doctor and nursing staff to ensure medications are monitored and administered safely to residents [28].

Errors Related to the Supply of Medication

The supply of medication to long-term care facilities is a complex process fraught with logistical difficulties. Since medications are usually supplied to long-term care facilities by off-site pharmacies, there is a problem with receiving medications in a timely manner. Often, the delivery of new or altered medications to a facility can take hours and, in some cases, days resulting in a missed dose, which essentially is a medication error [12]. This sort of delay and interruption to therapy can have a significant impact on the overall health and well-being of the resident concerned. Further, as is increasingly a common practice, if a long-term care facility uses Dose Administration Aids (DAAs) to administer medications to residents, then issues with supply become even more problematic.

DAAs are prepackaged medication systems with individual doses of either a day's supply or a weekly supply of medication arranged according to the dosage and regimen prescribed by a resident's treating doctor. A community pharmacist fills and dispenses medication into these packages either in a blister-type pack, a plastic sachet or a dosette-type container. A review of Australian studies of medication administration errors revealed that errors occurred in 15–20% of drug administrations when ward stock systems were used and dropped to 5–8% when individual patient systems were used [43]. These findings were compelling and provided the rationale for the introduction of DAAs into some long-term care facilities.

However, while these Australian studies showed that the rate of medication errors during administration has been reduced with the use of DAAs, there are other studies that show significant errors can occur with the packaging of these aids that could result in adverse outcomes for the recipients. Carruthers et al. [52] audited 42 residential aged care facilities to determine the accuracy of the packaging of DAAs and found that the rate of medication errors in DAA packaging was high. Results of the audit revealed substantial issues related to incorrect labelling, incorrect dose, incorrect dosage instructions, wrong medication dispensed, medications missing from a package and the supply of medication supplied that had been ceased by the treating doctor.

The recommendations from this study include the need to develop guidelines that addresses the supply of advanced packaging of medications. Additionally, regular audits (at least monthly) should be conducted in conjunction with the pharmacist and nursing staff.

Some DAA packaging systems have labels with images and descriptions of the medications contained within it. According to the manufacturer of one system, this feature is a safeguard as it could assist the staff to identify medication visually before administering [53]. However, a PCA or nurse should never assume that the picture and description on the DAA confirms that the medication in the container is in fact what was prescribed. In fact, any attempts to rationalise medications using this system could result in serious medication errors with very poor outcomes for the residents concerned.

Given that there are usually no doctors on-site in long-term care facilities, several phone calls to and from the doctor and the pharmacist who service the facility are required before any new medication is delivered. The pharmacist too is off-site and the medication chart needs to be photocopied and faxed to the pharmacy to confirm the requested alterations are valid. This can have serious consequences for the resident concerned as more often than not, a substantial amount of time elapses, sometimes hours, before the medication is delivered to the facility [54].

Moreover, should a resident from a long-term care facility visit a specialist at an outpatient clinic or be admitted to a hospital and then be discharged back to the facility, the process to ensure accurate and timely access to medication becomes even more complex. If the hospital dispenses medications in their original packaging for a resident returning to a facility where a DAA is in use, the medication cannot be administered until the treating doctor amends the medication chart to include the newly prescribed medication. The medication chart once again has to be photocopied and faxed to the pharmacy to confirm whether the requested alterations are valid before the supply is granted.

A multidisciplinary medication management committee can foster a co-operative environment for developing process improvement across the spectrum of medication management with the aim of reducing medication errors and improving resident outcomes. Regular audit and feedback coordinated by a multidisciplinary medication management committee can improve prescribing and administration practices [25]. Ensuring that the community pharmacy is represented on such a committee can help with improving the timeliness of medication supplies, to reduce pharmacy errors and to emphasise the importance of timely supply by using illustrative case studies [32].

Errors in Administration of Medication

Medication administration errors can be considered as: any difference between what the patient received and what the prescriber intended in the original order [28]. In long term care facilities, the processes involved in the overall management of medications presents significant barriers to staff and their ability to ensure that medications are delivered to the resident in a safe and timely manner [30]. In contrast to a hospital setting where there is ready access to doctors, pharmacists and the supply of medications, an extraordinary amount of time is spent in long-term care facilities communicating with doctors and pharmacists, before the medication is finally delivered to the facility. This makes the timely administration of medications to residents almost impossible in some cases.

Medication errors have been acknowledged as a persistent problem associated with nursing practice, and throughout the literature on the subject of medication errors, there are recurring themes associated with the cause and contributing factors involved in medication errors. The most commonly cited issues involve the systems or processes in place, environmental issues, equipment, and lack of suitably qualified staff, inadequate supplies and distractions while administering medications [19].

A failure by nurses to adhere to the five rights of medication administration (right medication, right dose, right resident, right time, right route and given for the right reason) is commonly cited as contributing to the high incidence of medication errors [2, 32, 44, 55]. Cohen et al. [56] in their analysis of a survey to investigate nurses' attitudes and experiences regarding medication administration and error reporting found that nurses did acknowledge some failure in adhering to the "five rights" of medication administration. However, they did identify several external barriers that impacted on their ability to conscientiously adhere to the five rights of medication administration. Issues such as lack of appropriately qualified staff, interruptions during administration of medications, time spent securing supplies, attending to visiting doctors, and telephone calls were cited as impacting on their ability to administer medications safely.

Wrong Time

The administration of medication in long-term care facilities is further complicated because of limited human resources. In the hospital setting, there may be at least one nurse to five patients [33]. In a long-term care facility, it is not unusual to find only one Div 1 RN. The rest of the staff is made up of Div 2 RNs who may be endorsed to administer medications and PCAs with little or no formal training in medication management. Further, in long-term care facilities that provide low care to residents, it is not unusual for a PCA to be responsible for the administration of medications to residents.

Medication management in long-term care facilities is a time-consuming process with a high number of daily medications being given to residents who are dependent on staff for assistance to take their medications. It has been suggested that the systemic conditions, which lead to medication errors consist largely of workload, particularly medication workload in facilities where there are few nursing staff responsible for the administration of large numbers of medications to a large number of residents. In such conditions, the likelihood of medication errors occurring is increased [32].

This is supported in the findings of Young et al. [57]. In their study, they found that as many as 375 medications were administered by one staff member to 49 residents during a single morning medication round. Further, and not surprisingly, they found that in a 2 h observational period, the most common type of medication error was related to timeliness where approximately 70% of medications were administered to residents more than 1 h before or after the scheduled time.

Paradiso et al. [58] in their study noted a wide complexity of practices that nurses were engaged in during a medication round. For example, during a medication round nurses also: answered telephone enquiries, directed care-worker activities, dealt with residents' problems, attended to visiting doctors and managed staffing issues for future shifts.

Whether medications are administered either one hour before or after the scheduled time is a significant problem that depends on the type of medication involved and the health status of residents. While the literature on the impact of time and the administration of medication in long-term care facilities is sparse, there is no question that some medications, for example, insulin and antibiotics must be given at predetermined and regular times to ensure that therapeutic efficacy is maximised. The timing of the administration of medications has been identified in the literature as an issue in long term care facilities. Deans [53] found that nurses did not consider reporting medication given an hour late as a medication error and found that nurses were more likely to report a medication error when they believed patient safety may have been compromised.

Dickens et al. [44] report the findings of their study in a facility that used "runners" to assist in the administration of medication; runners were either another registered nurse or a personal care worker delegated to administer medications to specific residents by the nurse preparing them. Although the use of runners may have helped reduce the workload placed on one individual, the medication error rate in this study was found to be high. An error occurred in one in every five doses of medication administered. However, almost all medication errors occurred during the preparation stage with the most common error being that of an unauthorised dose form, such as, crushing modified release tablets or opening capsules to ease administration.

Wrong Dose

Errors in calculating the correct dose of medication is a problem for nurses and doctors alike, and several studies have identified that medication errors can result from the poor mathematical skills of both nurses and doctors [59–64]. Oldridge et al. [58] conducted a pilot study comparing doctors' abilities with those of other health-care professionals who are directly involved with drug dose calculations. They asked five questions related to drug calculations and their findings showed that overall, drug dose calculations were performed poorly with less than 14% of the participants answering all five questions correctly.

Nurses have given their support to continuing education on medication management and are forthcoming in identifying gaps in their knowledge about medications generally and highlight drug calculations in particular [42, 44]. Despite the argument that a change in knowledge does not necessarily produce a change in practice or that tests and continuing education on medication calculations does not reduce medication errors [38, 65], education in medication management should still be undertaken by all the staff responsible for the administration of medication to residents. It has been shown that inadequate drug information and outdated or limited references is a common contributing cause of medication errors [66].

The Nurses' Board of Tasmania [4] views continuing education as a preventative approach to improving medication safety, and it recommends testing nurses' knowledge of medications and medication calculations during their orientation period, or through in service updates, or by implementing policy requiring all nurses and staff involved in the administration of medications to complete an annual competency assessment. Also, Pepper and Towsley [67] did find some studies that demonstrated educational interventions consisting of academic detailing may be effective in improving prescribing practices and resident outcomes.

Altered Dose Forms

The practice of altering dose forms of medication long-term facilities is common [68]. Many older people in long-term care facilities have their medication altered for ease of administration [57]. Paradiso et al. [67] in their study of ten long-term care facilities observed that 34% of the medication was altered, that is, crushed and mixed with jam, custard or fruit prior to administration. While this practice aims to ensure residents do receive necessary medication, this practice raises many possible problems. Altering the formulation of a medication may cause increased toxicity, decreased efficacy, local irritant effects, unpalatability as well as rendering the medication unstable. For example, crushing sustained release or controlled release products can influence the rate of absorption and consequently lead to higher peak blood concentrations with a potential for the development of toxic effects. Crushing medication might also be considered unlicensed practice [69].

Before altering any medication, a check should be made with the pharmacist to determine whether an alternative formulation is available such as a dispersible or liquid form of the same medication. A list of medications should be made available from the pharmacist that identifies what medications can and cannot be crushed with instructions on how best to prepare for administration. If prescribed medications are unable to be altered, then the treating doctor needs to be informed so that he or she can reconsider the drug order.

If there is no alternative available, then information related to the best method of preparing the medication should be available. It has been suggested that tablets should be crushed first, then any capsules opened with the powder or granules are mixed gently using either pureed fruit or yoghurt to maximise the stability of the medication, to reduce the potential for irritant effects and to make it more palatable [57].

To reduce the potential for toxicity occurring during the preparation stage of crushing medications, it is important to cleanse the receptacle used to crush the medications between residents to ensure all previous medication is cleared from the device prior to use.

Residents who are unable to swallow medications in the form prescribed should have an assessment conducted by a speech pathologist to identify the underlying problem and the most appropriate strategies to assist with medication administration.

Wrong Resident

Unlike the hospital setting, where a nurse can identify and verify patients at the bedside by checking their identification bracelet with the unit record number on the medication chart, in long-term care facilities, identifying and verifying the right resident can be difficult. Long-term care facilities do not use identification bracelets and generally rely on a photograph placed on the front of the medication chart to identify a resident. To ensure medication is administered to the right resident requires a high quality photograph that captures an accurate and current image of the resident that leaves no doubt that the resident has been correctly identified.

One solution implemented in a long-term care facility to reduce problems with identification of residents is the use of identification in the form of jewellery. A range of sterling silver jewellery specially made to suit each resident was provided and engraved with the resident's name to provide a form of identification [67]. This not only maintains the resident's dignity, but also enhances safety during the administration of medication as it assists new staff or agency nurses to correctly identify residents prior to administering their medication.

Long-term care facilities are often quite (necessarily) explicit in their philosophy of care, which values resident choice, privacy and independence. This often involves negotiation with residents to strike a balance between freedom, autonomy and the potential risks for themselves, other residents and staff. Residents in long-term care facilities who choose to self administer their medications are required to demonstrate their understanding and competence to do so. While a resident may be considered competent to self administer, this can be problematic in a facility that does not have a secure, locked drawer or cabinet where medications can be stored. A robust system of managing and storing medications for those residents who are self administering needs to be in place to ensure the safety of other residents who may inadvertently take medications not prescribed for them and to maintain a resident's independence and control.

Other residents may request that their medications be placed on an over bed table or locker so that they can take them when they choose to do so. This too is problematic, because an essential part of the administration process is to witness or assist the resident to physically take the medication prior to signing that the medication has, in fact, been administered as prescribed. To do otherwise could be viewed as a serious breach of professional codes of conduct.

Conclusion

Medication management in long-term care settings is a complex process confounded by the very nature of the setting. As has been discussed, across the whole continuum of medication management from the prescription, supply, and finally administration of medication, errors are common and similar to those that occur in other settings. There is little robust data on the incidence and prevalence of medication errors in long-term care settings and on interventions that successfully reduce the error rate. While medication errors, types, causes and contributing factors have been extensively studied in hospital settings, well-designed research studies that focus specifically on medication errors in long-term care settings are seriously lacking.

The issues that are peculiar to long-term care settings such as the staffing profile, use of DAAs, the practice of altering dose forms of medication, delays in supply, and the lack of onsite pharmacy and medical staff all serve to generate a more complex series of events that contribute to the occurrence of medication errors. Further research to clearly identify the best approaches to reduce medication errors in long term care settings is well overdue.

References

1. Patient Safety Solutions (2007) Patient safety & quality healthcare. Lionheart, USA
2. Banning M (2007) Medication management in care of older people. Wiley, UK
3. Nebeker JR, Barach P, Samore MH (2004) Clarifying adverse drug events: a clinician's guide to terminology, documentation, and reporting. Ann Intern Med 140:795–801
4. Pepper GA, Towsley GL (2007) Medication errors in nursing homes: incidence and reduction strategies. J Pharmaceut Finance Econ Policy 16:5–133
5. Safety of Medicines (2002) A guide to detecting and reporting adverse drug reactions. World Health Organization, Geneva. http://www.who.int/medicines/. Accessed 10 June 2008
6. Medication Safety in Australia (2008) Current status at November 2007. National Prescribing Service, Sydney, Discussion paper
7. Roughead EE, Barratt JD, Gilbert AL (2004) Medication-related problems commonly occurring in an Australian community setting. Pharmacoepidemiol Drug Saf 13:83–87
8. Burgess CL, D'Arcy C, Holman J, Satti AG (2005) Adverse drug reactions in older Australians, 1981–2002. Med J Aust 182:267–270
9. National Prescribing Service (2006) Indicators of quality prescribing in Australian general practice. A manual for users. National Prescribing Service Limited, Sydney, Australia
10. Routledge PA, O'Mahony MS, Woodhouse KW (2003) Adverse drug reactions in elderly patients. Br J Clin Pharmacol 57:121–126
11. Mannesse CK, Derkx FHM, De Ridder MA, Man AJ, Van Der Cammen TJM (2000) Contribution of adverse drug reactions to hospital admission of older patients. Age Ageing 29:35–39

12. Runciman WB, Roughead EE, Semple SJ, Adams RJ (2003) Adverse drug events and medication errors in Australia. Int J Qual Health Care 15:49–59
13. Classen S, Mann W, Wu SS, Tomita MR (2004) Relationship of number of medications to functional status, health, and quality of life for the frail home-based older adult. OTJR 24:151–160
14. Banning M (2005) Medication management: older people and nursing. Nurs Older People 17:20–23
15. Ballentine N (2008) Polypharmacy in the elderly maximizing benefit, minimizing harm. Crit Care Nurs Q 31:40–45
16. Salam A, Mandal S, Kumar A, Almula AA (2008) Polypharmacy: cure or curse? Qual Ageing 9:24–28
17. Laroche LM, Charmes JP, Nouaille Y, Picard N, Merle L (2006) Is inappropriate medication use a major cause of adverse drug reactions in the elderly? Br J Clin Pharmacol 63:177–186
18. George J, Munro K, Mc Caig D, Stewart D (2006) Risk factors for medication misadventure among residents in sheltered housing complexes. Br J Clin Pharmacol 63:171–176
19. Furniss L, Craig SKL, Burns A (1998) Medication use in nursing homes for elderly people. Int J Geriat Psychiatry 13:433–439
20. Gilbert AL, Roughead EE, Beilby J, Mott K, Barratt JB (2002) Collaborative medication management services: improving patient care. Med J Aust 177:189–192
21. Griffiths R, Johnson M, Piper M, Langdon R (2004) A nursing intervention for the quality use of medicines by elderly community clients. Int J Nurs Pract 10:166–176
22. Cox-Curry L, Walker C, Hogstel MO, Burns P (2005) Teaching older adults to self-manage medications preventing adverse drug reactions. J Gerontol Nurs 31:32–42
23. Snowdon J, Day S, Baker W (2006) Audits of medication use in Sydney nursing homes. Age Ageing 35:403–408
24. Department of Health and Ageing (2006) Aged care in Australia. Commonwealth of Australia, Canberra
25. Australian Pharmaceutical Advisory Council (2002) Guidelines for medication management in residential aged-care facilities, 3rd edn. Commonwealth of Australia, Canberra
26. Beya SC (2005) Best practices for safe medication administration. AORN 81:895–898
27. Pape TS, Guerra DM, Muzquiz M, Bryant JB et al (2005) Innovative approaches to reducing nurses' distractions during medication administration. J Contin Educ Nurs 36:108–116
28. Vogelsmeier A, Scott-Cawiezell J, Zellmer D (2007) Barriers to safe medication administration in the nursing home: exploring staff perceptions and concerns about the medication use process. J Gerontol Nurs 33:5–12
29. Pelleteir P (2001) Medication errors: a lesson from long-term care. Nurs Manage 32:49–50
30. McBride-Henry K, Foureur M (2007) A secondary care nursing perspective on medication administration safety. J Adv Nurs 60:58–66
31. Nichols P, Copeland TS, Craig IA, Hopkins P, Bruce DG (2008) Learning from error: identifying contributory causes of medication errors in an Australian hospital. Med J Aust 188:276–279
32. Young HM, Gray SL, McCormick WC, Sikma SK, Reinhard S, Tripett LJ et al (2008) Types, prevalence, and potential clinical significance of medication administration errors in assisted living. J Am Geriatr Soc, Early view. http://0www3.interscience.wiley.com. Accessed 10 June 2008
33. Baker H (1996) Australian nursing practice and the quality use of medicines. Royal College of Nursing, Australia, Discussion paper no. 3
34. Chassin MR, Becher EC (2002) The wrong patient. Ann Intern Med 136:826–833
35. Barker KN, Flynn EA, Pepper GA, Bates DW, Mikeal RL (2002) Medication errors observed in 36 health care facilities. Arch Intern Med 162:1897–1903
36. Curtis LH, Ostbye T, Sendersky V, Hutchison S, Dans PE, Wright A, Woosley RL, Schulman KA (2004) Inappropriate prescribing for elderly americans in a large outpatient population. Arch Intern Med 164:1621–1625

37. Howard R, Avery T (2004) Inappropriate prescribing in older people. Age Ageing 33:530–532
38. Jenkins RH, Vaida AJ (2007) Simple strategies to avoid medication errors. Fam Pract Manag 14:41–47
39. Beers MH (1997) Explicit criteria for determining potentially inappropriate medication use by the elderly. An update. Arch Intern Med 157:1531–1536
40. Budnitz DS, Sheabab N, Kegler SR, Richards L (2007) Medication use leading to emergency department visits for adverse drug events in older adults. Ann Intern Med 147:755–765
41. Gurwitz JH, Field TS, Judge J, Rochon P, Harrold LR, Cadoret C, Lee M, White K, La Prinob J, Erramuspe-Mainard J, De Florio M, Gavendo L, Auger J, Bates DW (2005) The incidence of adverse drug events in two large academic long-term care facilities. Am J Med 118:251–258
42. Tang FI, Sheu SJ, Yu S, Wei IL, Chen CL (2007) Nurses relate the contributing factors involved in medication errors. J Clin Nurs 16:447–457
43. Carruthers A, Naughton K, Mallarkey K (2008) Accuracy of packaging of dose administration aids in regional aged care facilities in the Hunter area of New South Wales. Med J Aust 188:280–282
44. O'Shea E (1999) Factors contributing to medication errors: a literature review. J Clin Nurs 8:496–504
45. Burns P, Dalley A (2007) The introduction of electronic medication charts and prescribing in aged care facilities: an evaluation. Australas J Ageing 26:131–134
46. Bomba D, Land T (2006) The feasibility of implementing an electronic prescribing decision support system: a case study of an Australian public hospital. Aust Health Rev 30:380–388
47. Strohecker S (2003) Polished automation tools allow patient safety to shine. Nurs Manag 34:34–37
48. Institute for Safe Medication Practices (2007). ISMP's list of high-alert medications. http://www.ismp.org/Tools/highalertmedications.pdf. Accessed 10 June 2008
49. Thompson A (2004) Why do therapeutic drug monitoring. Pharmaceut J 273:153–155
50. Benbow D (2008) Why do drug errors happen? Texas Board Nurs Bull 39:6–7
51. Australian Pharmaceutical Advisory Council (2000) Integrated best practice model for medication management in residential aged care facilities, 2nd edn. Commonwealth Department of Health and Aged Care, Canberra
52. Webstercare Medication Pak. http://www.webstercare.com.au/team.asp. Accessed 20 July 2008
53. Dickens G, Stubbs J, Haws C (2008) Delegation of medication administration: an exploratory study. Nurs Stand 22:35–40
54. Roberts MS, Stokes JA, King MA, Lynne TA, Purdie DM, Glasziou PP et al (2001) Outcomes of a randomized controlled trial of a clinical pharmacy intervention in 52 nursing homes. J Clin Pharmacol 51:257–265
55. Cohen H, Robinson ES, Mandrack M (2003) Getting to the root of medication errors: survey results. Nursing 33:36–45
56. Gerdtz MF, Nelson S (2007) 5–20: A model of minimum nurse-to-patient ratios in Victoria. Aust J Nurs Manag 15:64–71
57. Paradiso LM, Roughead EE, Gilbert AL, Cosh D, Nation RL, Barnes L, Cheek J, Ballantyne A (2002) Crushing or altering medications: what's happening in residential aged-care facilities? Australas J Ageing 21:123–127
58. Deans C (2005) Medication errors and professional practice of registered nurses. Collegian 12:29–33
59. Antonow JA, Smith AB, Silver MP (2000) Medication error reporting: a survey of nursing staff. J Nurs Care Qual 15:42–48
60. Wright K (2008) Drug calculations part 1: a critique of the formula used by nurses. Nurs Stand 22:40–42
61. Warburton P, Kahn P (2007) Improving the numeracy skills of nurse prescribers. Nurs Stand 21:40–43

62. Wheeler DW, Wheeler SJ, Ringrose TR (2007) Factors influencing doctors' ability to calculate drug doses correctly. Int J Clin Pract 6:89–94
63. Harding L, Petrick T (2008) Nursing student medication errors: a retrospective review. J Nurs Educ 47:43–47
64. Oldridge GJ, Gray KM, Mc Dermott LM, Kirkpatrick CMJ (2004) Pilot study to determine the ability of health-care professionals to undertake drug dose calculations. J Intern Med 34:316–319
65. Dennison RD (2007) A medication safety education program to reduce the risk of harm caused by medication errors. J Contin Educ Nurs 38:176–184
66. Standards of medication management for nurses and midwives (2008). The Nurses Board of Tasmania, Australia
67. Gowan J (2006) The northern division of medical practice. Div News 16:18–19
68. Barnes L, Cheek J, Nation RL, Gilbert A, Paradiso L, Ballantyne A (2006) ISMP's list of high-alert medications. J Adv Nurs 56:190–199
69. Harulow S (2003) Security jewellery: an answer to an age-old problem? Australas Nurs J 10:27

The Impact of Medication on Nutritional Status of Older People

Yvonne Coleman

Keywords Drug–nutrient interactions • Drug–food interactions • Medications and nutrition in older people

Ageing and Nutrition

The connections between diet, health and disease are relevant to older people. Inappropriate dietary intake is a significant contributor to both chronic and acute morbidity, and illness itself affects food intake and compromises resistance to disease. Older people are at greater risk than other age groups of marginal nutritional status and are at higher risk of nutritional deficiency in times of stress or health problems [1, 2].

As one becomes older, the physiology changes and may require "assistance" to maintain status; examples of areas in which such changes may occur include blood pressure, heart function, bladder control, diabetes and memory. Many pharmaceutical agents have been developed to "assist" the body in maintaining its physiologically desirable status. Turnheim [3] has published an excellent review on the pharmacokinetics (absorption, distribution, metabolism, excretion) and pharmacodynamics (clinical effects) of drugs in older people, and consequently only some aspects will be mentioned in this chapter.

The impact of medications on the nutritional status of older people confers both advantages and disadvantages. For simple health problems, the advantages are apparent – if a person

- is depressed and not eating, then the treatment of the depression will also result in improved food intake;

Y. Coleman (✉)
Nutrition Consultants Australia, Victoria 3122, Australia
e-mail: info@nutritionconsultantsaustralia.com.au

S. Koch et al. (eds.), *Medication Management in Older Adults:*
A Concise Guide for Clinicians, DOI 10.1007/978-1-60327-457-9_6,
© Springer Science+Business Media, LLC 2010

- has caught a bacterial germ, feels unwell and is not eating well, then treatment with an antibiotic will result in recovery from the infection and consequent improved food intake;
- has uncontrolled AF or CCF, then they do not feel well and consequently have a poor appetite. However, the appetite returns once the AF/CCF is controlled.

Ultimately, if a person is feeling unwell, he or she is more likely not to eat or to eat poorly. Once the cause of the unwellness is treated, typically with a drug, then the person feels better and the food intake improves naturally. The disadvantages of medications on nutritional health can be categorised into two main categories:

- Direct and indirect effects or costs
- Contributing factors

Direct and Indirect Effects or Costs

The costs of medication on nutritional status are not necessarily apparent and are quite extensive. This section of the chapter explores the potential direct and indirect effects of medications in older people.

Appetite

Direct effects of some drugs can significantly increase or decrease appetite. Both excessive and poor food intake have been found to manifest as health problems.

Indirect effects such as chronic side effects include nausea, vomiting, constipation, diarrhoea, altered sense of taste, dry mouth, drooling all of which exacerbate poor food intake. It is unlikely that older people will want to eat if they have chronic constipation, chronic diarrhoea, chronic nausea, or the food is tasteless, or has a bitter or metallic taste. If we accept that an individual should not be asked to tolerate chronic diarrhoea, chronic nausea or tasteless food, then we have a responsibility to ensure that the patient is provided appropriate care.

Absorption

The direct effects of drugs such as carbamazepine competitively inhibit biotin absorption [4–7]. Biotin deficiency symptoms include nausea, vomiting, anorexia, glossitis, pallor, depression, lassitude, substernal pain, scaly dermatitis, desquamation of the lips, as well as anaemia, muscle pains, hypercholesterolaemia or electrocardiograph abnormalities [8]. This cluster of symptoms does not readily lead one to consider a biotin deficiency, and consequently its treatment is overlooked.

There are many examples whereby concurrent administration of a mineral binds the active drug ingredient and results in decreased availability of both nutrient and drug; examples include iron and thyroxine [9], calcium and thyroxine [10], iron and levodopa [2].

The indirect effects on absorption can be seen in drugs such as proton pump inhibitors. The effects are associated with reduction in gastric acid secretion [11] resulting in potentially altered absorption dynamics of both drugs and nutrients that are pH sensitive.

Metabolism

Drugs, such as the phenothiazines, which are riboflavin (vitamin B2) derivatives [12], cause riboflavin deficiency by impairing the formation of flavin adenine dinucleotide (FAD) from riboflavin [13]. Riboflavin deficiency symptoms include cheilosis (lesions of the lips), angular stomatitis (angles of the mouth), glossitis (a fissured and magenta-coloured tongue), seborrhoeic follicular keratosis of the nose and forehead, dermatitis of the anogenital region and intense photophobia [8]. This cluster of symptoms does not readily lead one to consider a riboflavin deficiency, and consequently its treatment is overlooked.

Excretion

The impact on the excretion function of the body can be seen in drugs such as the loop diuretics, which increase urinary excretion of calcium [14], magnesium [14], potassium [14] and sodium [14, 15]. Digoxin increases urinary excretion of magnesium [16], while aspirin increases excretion of vitamin C [17]. Excepting potassium, there are no current standard management strategies to replace the other "lost" nutrients.

Weight

Weight either directly or indirectly influences drug dose calculations; therefore, as weight changes so should drug doses. The following scenario provides an example of this. Mrs X was an elderly, 90-kg lady admitted to a residential aged care facility with hypothyroidism as one of her diagnoses. Two years later, Mrs X weighed 45 kg; however, her thyroxine dose had not been adjusted as she lost weight and so she became overmedicated and was therefore unable to eat adequately to meet her increased body requirements.

Drug–Food Interactions

There is an increasing range of foodstuffs and food components with which drugs can or may interact. This can lead to confusion about the safety of foods in relation to prescribed drugs. Examples include cocoa and blood pressure [18, 19], salt and antihypertensives [20], high protein intake and warfarin [21].

Impaired Swallow Reflex

There is minimal advice for those with impaired swallow reflex and who require the prescribed drug(s), and there is no standard requirement for drug companies to make recommendations.

Enteral Feeds

Here too, there is minimal advice for those requiring enteral feeding and who require the prescribed drug(s), and there is no standard requirement for drug companies to make recommendations.

Change of Domicile

What is eaten and when it is eaten significantly changes when there is a change in domicile. This may include living alone to living with family or moving into a residential aged care facility, or hospital. Yet, it would appear that little regard is given to these changes and its impact on nutritional status.

Malnutrition

The plasma proteins (albumin, total proteins) are typically considered to be markers of nutritional status. Albumin is a primary transporter for a range of drugs including aspirin, furosemide, temazepam and thyroxine. Alteration to albumin status will result in alteration of drug availability and consequent effect. For example, hypoalbuminaemia will result in increased unbound warfarin and consequent increased INR.

Risk Classification

There is currently no classification system for categorising levels of risk associated with drug–nutrient and drug–food interactions [22]. Santos and Boullata [22] have proposed a classification system that includes interaction mechanism, significance of the interaction, severity of the interaction and recommendations to ameliorate the interaction.

Genser [23] comments "properly designed studies on the epidemiology of food-drug interactions and standardized management approaches and consensus toward specific drug-nutrient interactions are missing." There is a range of factors that contribute to the exclusion of drug impacts on nutritional health, including:

- Health professional training – the impact of medications on nutritional health is not addressed or is barely mentioned in the undergraduate training of doctors, nurses, pharmacist and dieticians.

  Santos and Boullata [22] comment that, excepting the well-described interactions, "drug-nutrient interactions are dismissed by many clinicians", and that it "is analogous to trivializing drug-drug interactions as nothing more than a tablet and a capsule binding together in the intestinal lumen and altering absorption".

- TGA Australia does not require testing of the nutritional consequences of drugs as part of the government approval process.

  Santos and Boullata [22] comment "to maximise a drug's benefit while minimizing adverse drug outcomes, it is necessary to recognize drug-nutrient interactions systematically as part of a drug regimen review."

- No generic term to categorise this neglected area or potential specialty.

  This author suggests that perhaps either pharmaconutrition or nutripharmacy would be suitable terms to encompass all the aspects of the impacts of medications on nutritional health, that is, drug–nutrient interactions, drug–food interactions and drug–nutrition interactions. Once a specialty is identified, then dedicated research would hopefully follow.

- No specific journal on the topic.

  The journal *Drug–Nutrient Interactions* ceased publication in the late 1980s; consequently, any research in this area is now published in a broad range of journals and is therefore difficult to access easily.

- Few publications on the topic.
  Recent publications include:

  Meckling KA (2006) Nutrient–drug interactions. CRC, Boca Raton
  Boullata JI, Armenti VT (2004) Handbook of drug–nutrient interactions. Humana, Totowa

McCabe BJ, Frankel EH, Wolfe JJ (2003) Handbook of food–drug interactions. CRC, Boca Raton

- Lack of readily accessible information for clinicians [22].
  There are only two publications that present the information in an easily accessibly format for clinicians:
  Coleman Y (2005) Drug–nutrient interactions the manual. Nutrition Consultants Australia, Melbourne
  Pronsky ZM (2008) Food medication interactions. Food–Medication Interactions, Birchrunville

- Over the counter (OTC) availability.

  Many nutrients, herbs and other health foods are readily available in pharmacies, health food shops and supermarkets; there are no warnings regarding potential interactions with prescribed drugs. Ernst [24] comments that there are both direct and indirect safety issues with herbs:

- Direct – as supplements, they are not required to meet with the same standard of regulatory compliance as prescription drugs;
- Indirect – the range of advice offered in self-help books and health food stores on the benefits of herbs has ranged from harmless to harmful.

Some Drug–Nutrient Interactions that could be Incorporated into Clinical Practice

Metformin and B12 Status

There is currently a scientific debate as to whether metformin does in fact cause or contribute to B12 deficiency. The debate and research findings will continue to remain confused until three issues are addressed:

a. Clearly defined cut-offs for B12 deficiency. That is, is a person diagnosed as deficient when there is clear pernicious anaemia or manifestations of more subtle B12 deficiency effects?
b. Whether the B12 deficiency markers (homocysteine, methylmalonic acid) and transcobalamin are more reliable markers of B12 status
c. When the acceptable pathology range for B12 status matches research findings

A simple management strategy that also short-circuits the debate would be regular calcium supplementation for all older people prescribed metformin. Bauman et al. [25] found that because ileal B12 absorption is calcium-dependent, calcium supplementation reverses the B12 malabsorption.

CCF and Furosemide

The combination of CCF and furosemide results in depletion of thiamine levels in a similar fashion to the depletion of potassium levels [26, 27]. While a potassium supplement is now prescribed, a thiamine supplement is not. Thiamine deficiency symptoms include anorexia, weight loss, gastrointestinal upset, peripheral and central neuropathy, muscle weakness, cardiovascular irregularities, as well as mental changes including loss of emotional control, paranoid trends, manic or depressive episodes and confusion [8]. This cluster of symptoms does not readily lead one to consider a thiamine deficiency, and consequently its treatment is overlooked. Since thiamine is important in cardiac function, it is possible that the prescription of furosemide may both heal and harm.

Digoxin Decreases Magnesium Levels

It is not standardised medical practice to check magnesium levels on a regular basis while digoxin is prescribed. Magnesium deficiency symptoms include confusion, disorientation, personality changes, loss of appetite, depression, muscle contractions and cramps, tingling, numbness, hypertension, abnormal heart rhythms, coronary spasm and seizures [28]. This cluster of symptoms does not readily lead one to consider a magnesium deficiency, and consequently its treatment is overlooked. Since magnesium is important in cardiac function both directly and indirectly (by converting thiamine to its active form), it is possible that the prescription of digoxin may both heal and harm.

Prednisolone May Deplete Chromium Status

Impaired glucose tolerance and diabetes are commonly associated with corticosteroid treatment [29]. Ravina et al. [29] investigated whether corticosteroid administration increased chromium losses, and whether steroid-induced diabetes could be reversed by supplemental chromium. The authors [29] found amelioration of steroid-induced diabetes in 51 of 54 cases tested, and a 50% reduction in the amount of drugs administered. They also found that a daily maintenance dose of 200 μg Cr/day was adequate to maintain ongoing euglycaemia.

If further investigations support these initial findings by Ravina et al. [29], then chromium supplementation may be a simple and effective management tool for the treatment of steroid-induced diabetes. Since there are no apparent contra-indications for the administration of chromium with the corticosteroids, then the two drugs could be administered at the same time. This would reduce confusion and therefore increase the likelihood of compliance in consumers of polypharmacy.

Conclusion

As consumers of more than 30% of all prescription drugs, older people are at particular risk of drugs impacting on their nutritional health [23]. The risk is increased because their changing physiology results in multiple co-morbidities that are treated with a variety of drugs and many nutritional aspects of polypharmacy have not been researched. There seems to be a number of issues that require redress before this burgeoning area of neglect is rectified and the results integrated into daily health care practice.

References

1. Shils ME, Olson JA, Shike M, Ross AC (eds) (1999) Modern nutrition in health and disease, 9th edn. Williams & Wilkins, Baltimore
2. Mason P (1994) Nutrition and dietary advice in the pharmacy. Blackwell, London
3. Turnheim K (2003) When drug therapy gets old: pharmacokinetics and pharmacodynamics in the elderly. Exp Gerontol 38:843–853
4. Rathman SC, Eisenschenk S, McMahon RJ (2002) The abundance and function of biotin-dependent enzymes are reduced in rats chronically administered carbamazepine. J Nutr 132:3405–3410
5. Said HM, Redha R, Nylander W (1989) Biotin transport in the human intestine: inhibition by anticonvulsant drugs. Am J Clin Nutr 49:127–131
6. McMahon RJ (2002) Biotin in metabolism and molecular biology. Annu Rev Nutr 22:221–239
7. Said HM (1999) Cellular uptake of biotin: mechanisms and regulation. J Nutr 129:490S–493S
8. Ball GFM (2004) Vitamins their role in the human body. Blackwell, Oxford
9. Campbell NRC, Hasinoff BB, Stalts H, Rao B, Wong NCW (1992) Ferrous sulfate reduces thyroxine efficacy in patients with hypothyroidism. Ann Intern Med 117(12):1010–1013
10. Singh N, Singh PN, Hershman JM (2000) Effect of calcium carbonate on the absorption of levothyroxine. JAMA 283(21):2822–2825
11. Mason P (1994) Nutrition and Dietary Advice in the Pharmacy. Blackwell Scientific Publications: London
12. Paiva SAR, Sepe TE, Booth SL, Camilo ME, O'Brien ME, Davidson KW, Sadowski A, Russell RM (1998) Interaction between vitamin K nutriture and bacterial overgrowth hypochlorhydria induced by omeprazole. Am J Clin Nutr 68:699–704
13. McCabe BJ, Frankel EH, Wolfe JJ (2003) Handbook of food-drug interactions. CRC Press, Boca Raton
14. Pinto J, Huang YP, Rivlin RS (1981) Inhibition of riboflavin metabolism in rat tissues by chlorpromazine, imipramine, and amitriptyline. J Clin Investig 67:1500–1506
15. Cohen N, Golik A, Dishi V, Zaidenstein R, Weissgarten J, Averbukh Z, Modai D (1996) Effect of furosemide oral solution versus furosemide tablets on diuresis and electrolytes in patients with moderate congestive heart failure. Miner Electrolyte Metab 22:248–252
16. Sica DA (2004) Diuretic-related side effects: development and treatment. J Clin Hypertens 6(9):532–540
17. Cohen N, Almoznino-Sarafian D, Alon I, Gorelik O, Shteinshnaider M, Chachashvily S, Averbukh Z, Golik A, Chen-Levy Z, Modai D (2003) Serum magnesium aberrations in furosemide (frusemide) treated patients with congestive heart failure: pathophysiological correlates and prognostic evaluation. Heart 89:411–416

18. Smith CH (1995) Drug-food/food-drug interactions. In: Morley JE, Glick Z, Rubenstein LZ (eds) Geriatric nutrition, 2nd edn. Raven Press, New York, pp 311–328

19. Taubert D, Roesen R, Schomig E (2007) Effect of cocoa and tea intake on blood pressure. Arch Intern Med 167:626–634

20. Taubert D, Roesen R, Lehmann C, Jung N, Schomig E (2008) Effects of low habitual cocoa intake on blood pressure and bioactive nitric oxide. JAMA 298(1):49–60

21. Darbar D, Fromm MF, Dell'Orto S, Kim RB, Kroemer HK, Eichelbaum M, Roden DM (1998) Modulation by dietary salt of verapamil disposition in humans. Circulation 98:2702–2708

22. Hornsby LB, Hester EK, Donaldson AR (2008) Potential interaction between warfarin and high dietary protein intake. Pharmacotherapy 28(4):536–539

23. Santos CA, Boullata JI (2005) An approach to evaluating drug-nutrient interactions. Pharmacotherapy 25(12):1789–1800

24. Genser D (2008) Food and drug interaction; consequences for the nutrition/health status. Ann Nutr Metab 52(Suppl 1):29–32

25. Ernst E (1998) Harmless herbs? A review of the recent literature. Am J Med 104:170–178

26. Bauman WA, Shaw W, Jayatilleke E, Spungen AM, Herbert V (2000) Increased intake of calcium reverses vitamin B12 malabsorption induced by metformin. Diabetes Care 23:1227–1231

27. Rieck J, Halkin H, Almog S, Seligman H, Lubetsky A, Olchovsky D, Ezra D (1999) Urinary loss of thiamine is increased by low doses of furosemide in healthy volunteers. J Lab Clin Med 134:238–243

28. Suter PM, Vetter W (2000) Diuretics and vitamin B1: are diuretics a risk factor for thiamin malnutrition? Nutr Rev 58(10):319–323

29. Kohlmeier M (2003) Nutrient metabolism. Academic, Amsterdam

30. Ravina A, Slezak L, Mirsky N, Bryden NA, Anderson RA (1999) Reversal of corticosteroid-induced diabetes mellitus with supplemental chromium. Diabet Med 16:164–167

Medication Management in Older Adults: What a Systematic Review Tells Us

Brent Hodgkinson

Keywords Medication errors • Aged • Prescriptions • Drug • Adverse event • Elderly • Adults • Drugs • Medication • Systematic review

What the Literature Says

An adverse drug event (ADE) can be defined as harm that can result from the nature of the drug (classed as an adverse drug reaction or ADR) or harm that results from the manufacture, distribution or use of medicines [1].

In Australia, around 59% of the general population uses prescription medication with this number increasing to about 86% in those aged 65 and over, and with 83% of the population over 85 using two or more medications simultaneously [2]. A recent study suggests that between 1.6% of all hospital admissions in Australia were associated with ADE, with 43% of these events deemed preventable [1]. In a recent review in the U.S, 27.6% of ADE in older persons in an ambulatory setting were determined to be preventable [3]. The Harvard Medical Practice study in the United States found that in hospital patients disabled by some form of medical treatment, 19% of recorded adverse events were related to medications [4]. Older Australians have higher rates of medication incidents due to higher levels of medicine intake and increased likelihood of being admitted to hospital (hospital statistics being the main source of medication incident reporting) [5]. In the community setting, it has been estimated that up to 400,000 ADEs may be managed in general practices each year in Australia [5]. In both public and private acute care hospitals, ADRs have been implicated in 27% of all recorded deaths [1]. The financial burden is also staggering with one estimate putting the cost of preventable medication

B. Hodgkinson (✉)
BlueCare, PO Box 1539, Milton BC, QLD 4064, Australia
e-mail: b.hodgkinson@bluecare.org.au

S. Koch et al. (eds.), *Medication Management in Older Adults:*
A Concise Guide for Clinicians, DOI 10.1007/978-1-60327-457-9_7,
© Springer Science+Business Media, LLC 2010

errors the US alone between \$17 and \$29 billion per year [6]. In Australia, the cost has been estimated at over \$350 million annually [7].

As medication errors can occur at all stages in the medication process, from prescription by physicians to delivery of medication to the patient by nurses, and in any site in the health system, it is essential that interventions be targeted at all aspects of medication delivery [5].

What Are the Types and Causes of Medication Errors?

In a recent American review of ADEs in older persons in an ambulatory setting, the most common ADEs were errors in prescribing (58.4%) and monitoring (60.8%) [3]. Monitoring errors were largely due to a failure to act on information from clinical findings or laboratory results. The authors also found that patient adherence was a mitigating factor in many ADE.

This is reflected in a recent review by the Australian Council for Safety and Quality in Health Care; the types of medication errors most frequently encountered in an Australian health care setting and their likely causes was reported [5].

Errors in Hospital

The most common errors related to medication that are encountered in hospitals in Australia are:

1. Prescription/medication ordering errors
2. Dispensing errors
3. Errors in administration of medicines
4. Errors in the medication record

Data from the Australian Incident Monitoring System showed that most medication incidents occurring in hospital were categorised as omissions (>25%), overdoses (20%), wrong medicines (10%), drug of addiction discrepancy (<5%), incorrect labelling (<5%) or an ADR (<5%). However, little is known as to why medication errors occur in Australian hospitals. Failure to read, or misreading the chart, and a lack of robust systems for prescribing and ordering were suggested as the reasons for most of these errors [5].

Errors can occur at any step in the medication process. A recent Australian review has attempted to describe the types of medication errors at each stage in the process [5].

Prescription/Medication Ordering Errors

Medication errors occur during the prescribing or interpretation/translation of orders from one document to another. Based on limited Australian data on prescription errors, approximately 2% of all prescriptions have the potential to cause an adverse event with the most common causes being the wrong or ambiguous dose, missing dose, or the directions for use were unclear or absent. This can be compared with other countries in which the medication error rates have been reported to be between 2 and 7% [8].

Dispensing Errors

Dispensing errors occurring within the hospital pharmacy have not been comprehensively studied. Error rates have been reported to range from 0.08 to 0.8% of all items dispensed. However, the causes and the potential for adverse events have not been reported [5].

Errors in Administration of Medicines

These errors occur when different patient medication supply systems are used.

When patients are given medicines from a common ward supply, error rates are between 15 and 20% compared with error rates of 5–8% when individual patient medicine supplies are provided [5].

Timing errors as high as 8% of administered doses has been shown to occur as a result of a patient being provided with a medicine at least 1 h before or 1 h after the scheduled time. These errors occur most likely due to time constraints and are unlikely to cause harm in the majority of cases [5].

Errors in the Medication Record

A common error is the lack of documentation of previous ADRs and allergies. Australian studies have found that previously known ADRs were not recorded in 75–77% of cases evaluated. In another study, 8% of cases had omissions of known allergic reactions in patient records. The causes and potential for ADEs were not described [5].

Errors in the Community Setting

In a recent study, the percentage of medication incidents resulting from the use of dose administration aids in residential aged care facilities in Australia reached 4.3% of all packs dispensed [9]. Reasons for incidents were missing medications from packs, wrong medication dispensed, supply of the wrong strength, incorrect labelling, pharmacy supplying medication already withdrawn by the GP, incorrect dosage instructions and medications not delivered to the facility.

Another review described medication incidents in general practice and community pharmacies [5]. General practitioners and pharmacists were asked to provide explanation as to why the medication incidents occurred.

General Practice

The types of medication incidents are described in Table 1.

The factors contributing to these errors, as described by doctors, are summarised in Table 2. *No correlation between these contributing factors and the resulting incident (Table 1), was made.*

Pharmacies

The most common types of dispensing errors reported by pharmacists are the selection of the incorrect strength, incorrect product or misinterpretation of a prescription. The major reason for selecting the incorrect strength or product has been described as the result of "look alike" or "sound alike" error.

Table 1 Types of medication errors in general medical practice

Type of incident	Rate per 100 incidents
Inappropriate drug	30
Prescribing error	22
Administration error	18
Inappropriate dose	15
Side effect	13
Allergic reaction	11
Dispensing error	10
Overdose	8
System inadequacies	7
Drug omitted or withheld	6

Source: [5, p. 33]

Table 2 Factors contributing to incidents in general practice

Contributing factor	Rate per 100 incidents
Poor communication between patient and health professionals	23
Action of others (not GP or patient)	23
Error of judgement	22
Poor communication between health professionals	19
Patient consulted other medical officer	15
Failure to recognise signs and symptoms	15
Patient's history not adequately reviewed	13
Omission of checking procedure	10
GP tired, rushed or running late	10
Patient misunderstood their problem and or treatment	10
Inadequate patient assessment	10

GP general practitioner
Source: [5, p. 33]

The report [5] describes an Australian survey of 209 community pharmacists where the major factors cited for contributing to dispensing errors were cited as:

- High prescription volume
- Overwork
- Fatigue
- Interruptions to dispensing
- "Look alike, sound alike" drug names

Other Factors That Contribute to Medication Errors

The review also described other possible factors that could contribute to medication error [5].

Inadequate Continuity of Care

Medication histories upon admission or discharge from hospital are often incomplete. Studies reviewing discharge prescriptions for patients found that 15% of medications intended to be continued were omitted at discharge, or that at least one medicine on average was omitted from the discharge prescription. At admission, one study found that on average one medicine was not documented on the medication history for every two patients.

In one survey of 106 general practitioners regarding the type of information they received from hospital about their patients, no notification was provided to the GP in over 50% of cases. Due to a change in patient medications by the hospital in 87% of cases, the patient's medicine at discharge was different to what the GP understood prior to admission in 72% of cases.

Finally, in a regional hospital in Queensland, of the referral medical records of 100 oncology patients, 72% had the potential for one or more errors in the patient's medication. The most common reasons for these errors were described as:

- Insufficient documentation to allow dosages to be confirmed
- Handwritten or illegible medication orders
- Lack of instruction about the length of time between cycles of chemotherapy

Multiple Health Care Providers

In one study of 204 people, 48% had medicines prescribed by more than one doctor and 28% had medicines dispensed by more than one pharmacy. The effect on medication error and ADEs has not been studied.

Keeping Unnecessary Medications

This involves keeping medications that are no longer in use or have passed their expiry date. In one small study where pharmacists made home visits to assist in medication management, 21% of people were keeping medicines that were no longer in use and 20% were keeping expired medications. The effect on medication error and ADEs has not been studied.

Generic Names/Trade Names

One study found that 29% of consumers did not understand the difference between the generic and trade name of a medication. Again, the effect on medication error and ADEs has not been studied.

Understanding the Label

In a single survey, 84% "older consumers" incorrectly interpreted the instruction to "take one tablet every 6 h, 1 h before food". The effect on medication error and ADEs has not been studied.

It is evident that the potential for an error in management of medication is substantial. But what according to the research literature are the most effective interventions to reduce the risk of medication errors in this population? A recent systematic review has evaluated the available literature in an attempt to answer this question [10].

The review followed the protocols described by the Cochrane Collaboration and the Joanna Briggs Institute. A protocol defining the inclusion criteria, search strategy, appraisal, data extraction and analysis methods was generated and followed.

What Interventions are Effective at Reducing Medication Errors in Older Persons?

Numerous reviews and research trials have attempted to answer this question. The original goal of this systematic review was to evaluate interventions to improve medication error incidence rates in an older population (≥65 years). However, the majority of studies did not direct interventions to this population, and therefore the evidence contained in this discussion is obtained largely from the general adult population. As persons aged 65 years and over account for a large proportion of admitted patients and 35% of all separations [11], it was considered appropriate to include studies from all clinical environments. As the review was intended to examine the effectiveness of specific interventions, studies that contained control groups were sought. A search of key words and words in the title and abstract such as "medication errors", "aged", "prescriptions", "drug", "adverse event", "elderly", "adults", "drugs" and "medication" was performed in the following databases:

- PubMed (NLM)
- Embase
- CINAHL (SilverPlatter)
- Current Contents
- Cochrane Library
- Science Citation Index Expanded
- ProceedingsFirst
- Social Science Index
- International Pharmaceuticals Abstracts

The appraisal of intervention studies was undertaken using a checklist developed by the Joanna Briggs Institute for Evidence Based Nursing and Midwifery.

Effectiveness

Numerous interventions to reduce the incidence of medication errors have been reported that evaluate all steps in the pathway of delivery of medication to the patient. Included in this review are evaluations of computerised ordering by physicians, drug order checking by pharmacists, supply and delivery of drugs to the respective medical units, and administration of drugs to the patients by nursing staff. Within each step of the process, different types of interventions were evaluated, such as the use of single versus double checking by nurses before administration of a drug, or the use of a dedicated nurse with a distinctive "jacket" to identify them as performing drug administration and not to be disturbed. Overall, however, for a number of the interventions discussed in this review, the level of evidence was low (small sample sizes, before and after studies) or the results were poorly reported or inconclusive. Another note of caution is that the definition and the severity of a medication error (e.g., life threatening vs minor), varied from trial to trial and was not always reported.

It was stressed in much of the research reviewed that medication errors do not necessarily translate into ADEs that could result in harm to patients. It was apparent from the literature that once a medication error was defined, the ease of determination of an error was dependent primarily on the level of reporting (i.e., the ease and willingness of clinicians to report an error). However, the resulting effect of a medication error, if any, on the patient was much harder to establish, and therefore many studies did not extend their outcomes to include this eventuality.

In several studies, the number of reported medication errors was actually seen to increase after implementation of an intervention. This may have been the result of increased vigilance and improved reporting systems rather than an increase in the incidence of errors. Therefore, in some studies, it was impossible to accurately determine the effectiveness of the specified intervention.

Computerised Systems

Computerised systems consisted of a variety of interventions including computerised physician ordering entry (CPOE), automated dispensing, bedside terminals, computer generated medication administration records (MAR), alert systems, and bar coding.

Computerised Physician Ordering Entry (CPOE) is described as a computer-based system whereby the physician writes all orders online. Within this system, the physician is provided with a menu of medications available from the formulary displayed with the default doses and a list of the potential range of doses. The system attempts to improve legibility, completeness and safety of orders. Clinical Decision Support Systems (CDSS) provides computerised advice on drug doses, routes and frequencies. CDSS can also perform drug allergy and drug–drug interaction checks as well as prompt for corollary orders (such as glucose levels after insulin has been ordered).

There was good evidence that CPOE systems combined with Clinical Decision Support Systems (CDSS) is effective in reducing medication errors in a general hospital population [8]. However, there was lower level evidence for the effectiveness of computer generated MAR, computer ADE detection and alerts. Finally, there was no evidence to suggest that the use of bedside terminal systems, or bar coding of patients or medications reduced medication error incidence, or that automated dosing systems reduced medication error incidence but only reduced errors in filling of dosing systems by technicians.

The majority of the research was in the use of CPOE to reduce medication errors and ultimately ADEs. While CPOE was shown to significantly decrease the incidence of medication errors, it was noted that there was little evidence for CPOE and/or CDSS reducing ADEs and actual patient harm [8].

A single report on the introduction of a computerised MAR reported only that medication errors deceased from 1 year to the next by 18% [12]. It was assumed from the report that medication errors were defined as a discrepancy between the MAR and the pharmacy order, but this was not implicitly stated. This single study does not unequivocally prove that it was effective at reducing medication errors as the change in medication errors was only compared from 1 year to the next. A positive of the new MAR was its readability over handwritten documents.

The use of a computer alert system in one study showed that in 44% of cases where the system alerted the physician to a potential risk of an ADE related injury, the physician was unaware of the risk [13]. This suggests that the system may be able to prevent a significant number of potentially harmful medical errors. However, the system consisted of only 37 drug specific ADEs and therefore would need to be expanded and updated to encompass a greater variety of risk.

Providing bedside terminal systems in one community hospital was evaluated for its effect on registered nurse time spent in direct care activities, overtime, attitudes toward the technology and unit medication error rate [14]. No difference in unit error rates was noted. However, the study duration for pre and post intervention observation was short at 40 h each and the errors were counted from reports on incident forms.

Identification of a single study in one systematic review [8] found that nurse use of bar codes in a point of care information system decreased the medication error rate in the hospital from 0.17% before the system was instituted to 0.05% after (p value not reported). While this result was encouraging, the use of the bar coding device was "easily and frequently circumvented", bringing into question the real contribution of the device to the overall error rate decrease. The reasons for this were not described.

However, a recent ethnographic study of nurse, physician, and pharmacist interaction with a newly instituted computerised system of bar code medication administration (BCMA) identified five negative themes (side effects) that may elucidate the reason for the under use of the bar-coding system reported in the review [15].

1. Nurse confusion over automated removal of medications by the BCMA.
2. Degraded coordination between the nursing staff and the physicians.
3. Nurses dropped activities to reduce workload during busy periods.
4. Increased prioritisation of monitored activities during busy periods.
5. Decreased ability to deviate from routine sequences.

The available evidence from a systematic review for the use of automated dispensing was found to be generally poor and did not support the suggestion that automated dispensing systems improved outcomes [8]. In a single study, the use of an auto-mated point-of-use dose system significantly reduced the rate of error in filling of dosage carts by technicians only [16].

Individual Patient Medication Supply

Individual medication supply systems have been shown to reduce medication error rates compared with other dispensing systems such as ward stock approaches. In Australian studies [17, 18], the use of individual patient supply was found to sig-nificantly reduce the medication error rate compared to a ward stock system of medication supply with studies showing a decrease in the medication error rate from 15.4% (76/494) to 4.8% (24/502), or missed medications from 5.7% (223/3,931 doses) to 4.1% (136/3,287 doses), respectively. However, one system-atic review suggested that the use of these systems shifts the chances for error from the nursing ward into the pharmacy, where distractions are also common and errors will occur [8].

Education and Training

Few studies were identified that examined the effectiveness of nursing education or training programs on the prevention of ADEs. From the two studies that were identified, there is no evidence to suggest that education addressing medication calculation, or a yearly medication examination are effective in reducing medica-tion errors [19, 20]. Looked at another way, neither written medication examina-tions nor education on medication calculation could improve nurse competence to prevent errors beyond the skills they had already accrued.

Pharmacists

There is evidence to suggest a role for clinical pharmacists in preventing ADEs in the inpatient setting. From a systematic review, intervention by a pharmacist in one study resulted in a 66% decrease in preventable ADEs due to medical ordering and a study of geriatric patients at the time of discharge found statistically significant decreases in medication errors [8]. From the same review, a randomised controlled trial (RCT) of 181 heart failure patients in the intervention group received clinical pharmacist evaluation, which included medication evaluation, therapeutic recom-mendations to the attending physician, patient education, and follow-up telemoni-toring. The control group received usual care. This study found all-cause mortality and heart failure events were significantly lower in the intervention group compared with the control group. The value of including a pharmacist during medication rounds was determined in two studies [21, 22]. Both studies displayed a decrease in the number of medication errors per 1,000 patient days with the improved availability of a pharmacist for consultation.

Evidence for the effectiveness of pharmacists in reducing ADEs in the outpatient setting is less compelling. In a recent systematic review evaluating the use of pharmacists in medication reviews to prevent emergency hospital admissions in older people (>60 years), there was no significant effect on all-cause admission or mortality [23]. However, a single study evaluated the process of reactive pharmacy intervention with the objective to identify prescriptions that may have defects to prevent a possible impact on the patient (i.e., an adverse event) [24]. The procedure was for the submitted prescription to be considered by the pharmacy prior to dispensing. If the prescription was considered defective, the pharmacist recorded the relevant drug details, a summary and categorisation of the problem, and the total time taken to initiate a response and resolve the problem. The study found that approximately 3% of prescriptions written over the period of 28 days were flagged as faulty. A high proportion of interventions were considered justified (83%) during the review, with 75% of interventions resulting in altered prescriptions.

Nursing Care Models

The strongest evidence suggests that having two nurses check medication orders prior to dispensing medication significantly reduces the incidence of medication errors [25]. However, the authors question the clinical advantage of this policy and do not recommend it. Weaker evidence suggested that single checking could be as safe as double checking, but was reliant on the number of medication errors *reported* in the medication incident records and may be a conservative estimate of the actual number of medication errors that actually occurred [26]. It has been demonstrated that the actual error rate could be 33% higher than reported rates [27].

There is no evidence to suggest that providing designated nurses to dispense medication significantly reduces the incidence of medication errors [14, 28, 29]. However, the use of the focused or Medsafe protocols in which nurses are identified as "not to be disturbed" can reduce distractions to nurses during medication administration [29]. Distractions were used as a surrogate measure of the potential for a medication error. While these strategies did not eliminate distractions during the medication "cycle", these interventions were shown to reduce them by as much as 87% compared with customary medication rounds. The weakness of this study may lie in the method of collection of distractions using a previously unvalidated collection tool and the unavoidable use of an unblinded observer.

Employment of a Medication Administration Review and Safety (MARS) committee was shown to have a positive effect on reducing the number of medication administration documentation errors over a period of 1 year [30]. This is likely due to the heightened awareness of medication error prevention and reporting.

There is limited evidence from one study to suggest that introducing the Partner in Patient Care (PIPC) model significantly reduces the incidence of medication errors [31]. This model was instituted in an attempt to reduce the workload on registered nurses by delegating less clinical tasks to a multi-skilled technician. Despite the claim that the PIPC model was effective at significantly reducing the medication error ratio (errors/patient day, $p = 0.008$), the data for before the institution of the PIPC model and after was not presented and therefore could not be verified.

As an example of the implementation of process change to improve the delivery of a specific drug and reduce the likelihood of an adverse event, diabetes education to nurses and the installation of blood glucose testing units in all wards were assessed [32]. Overall, the number of cases that received insulin within 60 min of a blood glucose test improved significantly. However, when individual units were evaluated, this improvement was not universal. Examination of time periods in which a significant reduction in time interval between time of blood glucose test and insulin administration was seen primarily for one but at only one time period in the other two. The unit showing greatest improvement showed consistently higher mean time intervals between blood glucose testing and insulin delivery during the control phase of the study at all measurement periods (means of 53–125 min) while the mean times of the other units were all below 60 min.

Conclusion

While the original goal of the systematic review was to evaluate interventions to improve medication error incidence rates in geriatric settings, it soon became apparent that little research had been performed strictly within this environment. However, as persons aged 55 years and above account for a large proportion of admitted patients and 51.7% of separations [33], it was considered appropriate to include studies from all clinical environments. Numerous interventions to reduce the incidence of medication errors were identified that evaluated all steps in the pathway of delivery of medication to the patient.

However, despite these relaxed inclusion criteria, it could be said that little empirical research could be identified for any single intervention. Most interventions were represented by no more than two or three trials using small sample sizes.

Of all the controlled trials identified, computerised systems were one of the most commonly tested interventions for the reduction of medication errors. There was good evidence that a CPOE system combined with CDSS can be effective in reducing medication errors in a general hospital population. However, other tested computerised systems such as computer generated MAR, computer ADE detection and alerts, bedside terminal systems, or bar coding of patients or medications provided little in the way of evidence for reducing medication error incidence.

Other than the computerised systems, the strongest evidence comes from research on the use of pharmacists to review medication orders in an inpatient setting. Some trials showed a benefit in reducing medication errors [8, 21, 22], all cause mortality or heart failure events [8].

For all other included research, the results do not definitively support their use to reduce medication errors or incidents. Even where some evidence is suggestive of effectiveness, such as research on individual patient medical supply suggesting decreases in error rates and missed medications [17, 18], the intervention on its own may not reduce the number of medication errors; but, as is argued by some, the intervention simply shifts the risk of error from the nursing ward back to the pharmacy [8]. Further, automated dosing systems were shown to reduce errors associated with filling of drawers by technicians but not to reduce overall medication error incidence. There is insufficient evidence to suggest any benefit of a pharmacist review of medications in an outpatient setting to reduce all cause admissions to emergency or to mortality [23]. However, a single study does suggest a role for the pharmacist as a check at the point of dispensing to identify potential faulty prescriptions [24].

It is surprising, given that, nursing staff have the final responsibility for the delivery of medication to patients and clients in both a clinical or residential setting that so few studies have assessed interventions at this stage of the medication process. Of the few studies that were identified, the evidence is less than compelling. Studies found that double checking of medication orders by nurses prior to administration of medicines did reduce medication error incidence [25], but it can be argued that this model would be very labour intensive and unrealistic in the community aged care nursing or residential aged care settings where one nurse per ward or per community client is the norm. This would also make the use of a dedicated nurse for medication administration [29] unfeasible despite the apparent reduction in distractions that may lead to reduced medication errors.

In essence then, in order to establish the effectiveness of most of the interventions reported in this review, more rigorously designed studies (e.g., randomised controlled trials) are necessary with larger participant numbers and longer trial periods.

However, it should be emphasised that the lack of evidence for the effectiveness of the reported interventions does not suggest that they are not effective but rather that limitations in trial design do not lead to any definitive answer to their effectiveness.

References

1. Runciman WB, Roughead EE, Semple SJ, Adams RJ (2003) Adverse drug events and medication errors in Australia. Int J Qual Health Care 15(Suppl 1):i49–i59
2. Australian Institute of Health and Welfare (2002) Older Australia at a glance, 3rd edn. AIHW & DOHA, Canberra, Report No.: AIHW Cat. No. AGE 25

3. Gurwitz JH, Field TS, Harrold LR et al (2003) Incidence and preventability of adverse drug events among older persons in the ambulatory setting. JAMA 289:1107–1116

4. Leape LL, Brennan TA, Laird N et al (1991) The nature of adverse events in hospitalized patients. Results of the Harvard Medical Practice Study II. N Engl J Med 324:377–384

5. Australian Council for Safety and Quality in Health Care (2002) Second national report on patient safety: improving medication safety. Australian Council for Safety and Quality in Health Care, Canberra

6. Strohecker S (2003) Medication management. Polished automation tools allow patient safety to shine. Nurs Manage 34: 34, 36, 38 passim

7. Roughead EE, Gilbert AL, Primrose JG, Sansom LN (1998) Drug-related hospital admissions: a review of Australian studies published 1988-1996. Med J Aust 168:405–408

8. Shojania KG, Duncan BW, MacDonald KM, Watchter RM (2001) A critical analysis of patient safety practices. Agency for Healthcare Research and Quality, Rockville, MD, Report No.: 43

9. Carruthers A, Naughton K, Mallarkey G (2008) Accuracy of packaging of dose administration aids in regional aged care facilities in the Hunter area of New South Wales. Med J Aust 188:280–282

10. Hodgkinson B, Koch S, Nay R, Nichols K (2006) Strategies to reduce medication errors with reference to older adults. Int J Evid Based Healthc 4:2–41

11. Australian Institute of Health and Welfare (2007) Older Australia at a glance. AIHW, Canberra

12. Adams C (1989) Computer-generated medication administration records. Nurs Manage 20:22–23

13. Raschke RA, Gollihare B, Wunderlich TA et al (1998) A computer alert system to prevent injury from adverse drug events: development and evaluation in a community teaching hospital. JAMA 280:1317–1320

14. Brown SJ, Cioffi MA, Schinella P, Shaw A (1995) Evaluation of the impact of a bedside terminal system in a rapidly changing community hospital. Comput Nurs 13:280–284

15. Patterson ES, Cook RI, Render ML (2002) Improving patient safety by identifying side effects from introducing bar coding in medication administration. J Am Med Inform Assoc 9:540–553

16. Ray MD, Aldrich LT, Lew PJ (1995) Experience with an automated point-of-use unit-dose drug distribution system. Hosp Pharm 30:18, 20–23, 27–30

17. Boyle CM, Maxwell DJ, Meguid SE, Ouaida D, Krass I (1998) Missed doses: an evaluation in two drug distribution systems. Aust J Hosp Pharm 28:413–416

18. McNally KM, Page MA, Sunderland VB (1997) Failure-mode and effects analysis in improving a drug distribution system. Am J Health Syst Pharm 54:171–177

19. Ludwig Beymer P, Czurylo KT, Gattuso MC, Hennessy KA, Ryan CJ (1990) The effect of testing on the reported incidence of medication errors in a medical center. J Contin Educ Nurs 21:11–17

20. Bayne T, Bindler R (1997) Effectiveness of medication calculation enhancement methods with nurses. J Nurs Staff Dev 13:293–301

21. Kucukarslan SN, Peters M, Mlynarek M, Nafziger DA (2003) Pharmacists on rounding teams reduce preventable adverse drug events in hospital general medicine units. Arch Intern Med 163:2014–2018

22. Shah NR, Emont AJ, Johnson VP (1994) Total quality management in action: pharmacy system changes to decrease medication incidents and increase clinical services. Hosp Pharm 29:676, 679–680

23. Holland R, Desborough J, Goodyer L, Hall S, Wright D, Loke YK (2008) Does pharmacist-led medication review help to reduce hospital admissions and deaths in older people? A systematic review and meta-analysis. Br J Clin Pharmacol 65:303–316

24. Hawkey CJ, Hodgson S, Norman A, Daneshmend TK, Garner ST (1990) Effect of reactive pharmacy intervention on quality of hospital prescribing. BMJ 300:986–990

25. Kruse H, Johnson A, O'Connell D, Clarke T (1992) Administering non-restricted medications in hospital: the implications and cost of using two nurses. Aust Clin Rev 12:77–83
26. Jarman H, Jacobs E, Zielinski V (2002) Medication study supports registered nurses' competence for single checking. Int J Nurs Pract 8:330–335
27. Larrabee JH, Ruckstuhl M, Salmons J, Smith L (1991) Interdisciplinary monitoring of medication errors in a nursing quality assurance program. J Nurs Qual Assur 5:69–78
28. Greengold NL, Shane R, Schneider P et al (2003) The impact of dedicated medication nurses on the medication administration error rate: a randomized controlled trial. Arch Intern Med 163:2359–2367
29. Pape TM (2003) Applying airline safety practices to medication administration. Medsurg Nurs 12:77–93, quiz 4
30. Schaubhut RM, Jones C (2000) A systems approach to medication error reduction. J Nurs Care Qual 14:13–27
31. Lengacher CA, Mabe PR, Bowling CD, Heinemann D, Kent K, Van Cott ML (1993) Redesigning nursing practice. The partners in patient care model. J Nurs Adm 23:31–37
32. Heatlie JM (2003) Reducing insulin medication errors: evaluation of a quality improvement initiative. J Nurses Staff Dev 19:92–98
33. Australian Institute of Health and Welfare (2008) Australian hospital statistics 2006–07. AIHW, Canberra

Misuse of Formulations in the Aged Care Setting

Andrew J. McLachlan and Iqbal Ramzan

Keywords Older people • Elderly • Ageing • Aging • Dose form alteration • Tablet crushing • Capsule opening • Stability • Dysphagia

Medicines and Older People

Other chapters in this book highlight the pattern of medication use in older people and the burden of unwanted effects. It is important to acknowledge that medicines play a key role in the treatment and prevention of illness in older people when they are appropriately used. The optimal use of medicines involves a complex interplay of factors [1]. Quality use of medicines underpins medication use in older people. Central to this concept is the use of medicines in a manner that is safe and effective. This concept not only includes the choice of an appropriate medicine and optimal dose selection but also a consideration of the most suitable dose form and the manner in which the medicines are stored and administered. These issues are articulated in the Australian Pharmaceutical Advisory Committee (APAC) guiding principles for medication management in the community [2] and residential aged care facilities [3]. Stubbs et al. [4] have highlighted that there are potential risks associated with dose form modification for both the patients and the staff.

The aim of this chapter is to discuss the key challenges related to dose form modification, identify how this can be achieved safely and how this contributes to quality use of medicines in older people. This chapter will also direct the reader to several resources to assist in achieving optimal medication use in older people [5].

A.J. McLachlan (✉)
Faculty of Pharmacy, University of Sydney and Centre for Education and Research on Ageing, Concord RG Hospital, Hospital Road, Concord, NSW 2139, Australia
e-mail: andrew.mclachlan@sydney.edu.au

S. Koch et al. (eds.), *Medication Management in Older Adults:*
A Concise Guide for Clinicians, DOI 10.1007/978-1-60327-457-9_8,
© Springer Science+Business Media, LLC 2010

Problems of Swallowing and Dose Form Modification

Swallowing difficulties (dysphagia) are common in stroke patients and in individuals with neurological conditions and is increasingly prevalent in ageing, leading to considerable problems in older patients [6–11]. Dysphagia can lead to significant effects on nutritional status, increases the risk of aspiration pneumonia and has significant effects on the quality of life [6]. Dysphagia is therefore relevant to the discussion in this chapter on the administration of solid medicines dose forms [6]. Patients with dysphagia are likely to receive crushed solid dose form medicines, which are added to thickening agents or soft foods, whereas patients with percutaneous endoscopic gastrostomy (PEG) or jejunostomy (PEJ) tubes receive crushed medicines added to an enteral feed [4].

A study by Wright [8] investigated medication administration practices by surveying 540 nursing staff employed in independent UK nursing homes. These data indicated that ~15% of residents had difficulty swallowing tablets and capsules and 61% ($n=331$) of nursing staff reported that they crushed or opened dose forms before administration. Interestingly, 88% of nurses reported that they identified and used liquid dose form alternatives in many of these patients. Taken together, these data indicate that dose form modification takes place in more than 80% of all UK nursing homes on at least a weekly basis [8]. These data are in agreement with practices in Australia and internationally [4]. Swallowing difficulties and other medication administration issues have a higher incidence in hospitalised older patients in acute settings [4, 6, 11]. Furthermore, older patients who are acutely ill are at a greatest risk of misadventure, and hence safe medication practice in this cohort is critical.

In patients with swallowing difficulties, appropriate assessment is essential. Quality use of medicines warrants a regular comprehensive reassessment of the need for all medicines in order to assess whether a temporary discontinuation for patients with swallowing difficulties is appropriate and safe. Careful consideration of alternative routes of administration is important.

Interventions to minimise the risks associated with dose form modification and improve such practices have focused on staff education and training to improve understanding of the clinical and pharmaceutical issues associated with dose form selection and modification [9, 10] and how these contribute to quality use of medicines [2, 3, 9]. In some countries (including Australia), pharmacists are accredited to conduct medication management reviews in older people at the risk of medication misadventure. These include Home Medicines Reviews (HMRs) and Residential Medication Management Reviews (RMMRs), which typically include a patient interview and therefore provide an excellent opportunity to identify patients who are having difficulties in swallowing and taking their medicines [2, 3]. Pharmacist-led medication reviews can identify individuals with perceived or actual swallowing difficulties and put strategies in place to ensure that dose form modification does not compromise safety and efficacy.

Dose Form Modification and the Risks for Older People

Different dose form modifications [4, 5, 12] include crushing solid dose forms (such as tablets), opening capsules, tablet splitting, reformulation of crushed tablets or capsule contents into a suspension, modifying (cutting) transdermal patches or changing the route of administration for which a formulation is usually designed. Table 1 highlights some examples of medicines that should not be modified and the risks associated with such modification.

Table 1 Examples of dose forms that should not be crushed (adapted from [22, 23] and other references in Table 2)

Dose form	Example	Comment
Enteric-coated tablets	Bisacodyl, enteric-coated aspirin, lansoprazole, omeprazole, pancrelipase, multiple erythromycin products	Modification of enteric-coated dose forms may render the active constituent inactive when it is directly exposed to the acidic and enzyme-rich environment of the gastric fluids
Extended or modified release tablets	Oxycodone or morphine extended release, diltiazem controlled dissolution, mesalamine, verapamil sustained release, oxybutynin extended release, tamsulosin, multiple theophylline products	These include dose forms designed to release the drug over an extended period of time, such as: 1. Multiple-layered tablets releasing drug as each layer is dissolved 2. Mixed release pellets that dissolve at different time intervals 3. Special matrices that are themselves inert, but slowly release drug from the matrix Crushing these tablets can lead to a significantly higher dose of drug over a shorter period with the risk of excessive pharmacological effects
Sublingual tablets	Sublingual nitrates (e.g. glyercyl trinitrate)	Sublingual dose forms are designed to dissolve quickly in oral fluids for rapid absorption by the abundant blood supply of the mouth Crushing and giving the contents of these tablets via the gastric route may render them ineffective due to extensive first pass metabolism

(continued)

Table 1 (continued)

Dose form	Example	Comment
Medicines with a bitter taste	Cefuroxime, ciprofloxacin, docusate, ibuprofen, hydroxychloroquine	Many medicines have a strong and unpalatable taste (hence the widespread use of film coating of tablets). Unmasking the strong taste can have a major impact on patient tolerability
Irritant medicines	Alendronate, atomoxetine, diflunisal, isotretinoin, piroxicam, risedronate, valproic acid	These medicines are examples of active ingredients, which are irritant to the oral, oesophageal or gastric mucosa. These medicines are typically presented in dose form or using dosing administration strategies, which minimise this risk. Modifying these dose forms has the potential to cause significant adverse effects in patients
Safety concerns	Finasteride, mycophenolate, other cancer chemotherapy agents	These medicines pose a health risk to healthcare professional who might handle them. These drugs are potentially carcinogenic, cytotoxic, mutagenic or teratogenic if handled without adequate protection or if aerosolised powder (generated during crushing) is inhaled. This is an Occupational Health and Safety concern for staff and carers handling and reformulating the drug. These medicines may be crushed but should always be handled and stored appropriately to minimise the risk of exposure to staff
Ability to stain teeth	Amoxicillin/clavulanate, linezolid, iron products	Some medicines and excipients (e.g. dyes) have the ability to discolour or stain teeth. This could have a major impact on patient experience and aesthetics

Altering the Route of Administration for Medicines

When a patient cannot swallow a medicine, it may be tempting to select an alternative formulation. For example, suitable alternatives might be the use of a liquid, trans-dermal, parenteral, buccal, sublingual, rectal or intranasal dose forms. When switching routes of administration in a given patient, consideration should be given to the relative bioavailability of the active ingredient and the need to alter dose regimens to maintain appropriate drug concentrations to elicit equivalent clinical outcomes. Rectal administration may be preferred under some circumstances but it should be noted that this route can lead to variability in both the rate and extent of drug absorption. High care patients may be administered medicines subcutaneously or intravenously where a suitable dose form exists; but this has significant patient care, staffing and cost implications, as well, challenges of venous access in older people. In some situations, clinicians may switch a patient to a therapeutically equivalent drug, which has a liquid dose form available. It is appropriate in these situations to use careful therapeutic monitoring. One scenario may be to use an intravenous formulation for oral or rectal administration. However, intravenous formulations are not always simple solutions and may contain other excipients (such as surfactants or alcohol) or have a pH, which is potentially irritant to mucosal tissues.

Dose Form Crushing

Crushing solid dose forms, which are not specifically designed for this, can have significant effects on drug pharmacokinetics, which in turn impacts on the drug therapeutic profile. This has the potential to result in poor efficacy and/or adverse effects (Table 1). Cleary et al. [13] investigated the impact of crushing extended release pentoxifylline tablets administered to healthy subjects when compared to intact tablets. They found that the time to maximum concentration (T_{max}) was shorter, the maximum plasma concentration (C_{max}) was higher and the increase in maximum plasma concentrations appeared to be associated with dose-related adverse effects [13]. Problems can also arise when crushed tablets interact with the food with which they are mixed; for example, food may bind to furosemide or calcium antagonists, keeping the drug in the gastrointestinal tract and decreases absorption [14, 15]. Crushing extended or modified release dose forms leads to risks of dose dumping and excessive effects (Table 1). Many dose forms are coated to mask a strong unpalatable taste, to protect the patient from mucosal irritation, to protect the medicine from gastric acid or to infer modified release characteristics (Table 1). Crushing such coated products destroys the coat.

The stability of pharmaceutical products is established and stringently evaluated in the final marketed packaging during drug registration. Once a dose form has been modified, there is no guarantee that the drug remains stable, and few published studies have evaluated drug stability in this setting. Immediate administration to patients when dose forms have been modified is therefore recommended.

Combining crushed tablet contents or the content of capsules carries risks of physicochemical incompatibility due to drug–drug or drug–excipient interactions. This has the potential to render active ingredients inactive or potentially toxic. An example is combining cations, such as iron or calcium, with medicines that have the potential to form insoluble chelate (e.g. bisphosphonates or tetracyclines) leading to insoluble complexes and a significant reduction in bioavailability.

Of greater concern when solid dose forms are crushed (or capsules opened) is the likely exposure of medicines or aerosolised powder to healthcare practitioners putting them at risk of adverse effects. This is particularly so when solid dose forms that contain cytotoxic, mutagenic or teratogenic medicines are modified (Table 1).

Administering Capsule Contents

Generally, capsule dose forms can be opened and the contents safely administered without further modification. Most capsules contain a simple mixture of powders (active and inert excipients) that may be dispersed in solution or soft food, if compatible with food constituents, and administered to patients. Some capsule contents should not be crushed as some modified release capsule dose forms contain intact modified release pellets, which would be disrupted if crushed. Encapsulation is also often used to mask bitter taste from unpalatable active ingredients/excipients. Care should be taken when opening capsule to account of this characteristic.

Modifying Transdermal Drug Delivery Systems

Transdermal drug delivery systems (TDDS) are increasingly used in the aged [16]. A challenge with these is the narrow range of drug delivery rates making it difficult to individualise drug dose. There are a range of TDDS that allow for effective transdermal absorption of drugs [17]. These include drug-reservoir type patches, which contain a saturated suspension of the drug in a water-miscible solvent homogeneously dispersed in a silicone elastomer matrix, a matrix-diffusion controlled transdermal system, a membrane-permeation controlled transdermal system and the gradient-charged transdermal systems [17]. One practice to individualise dose has been to use a cut portion of the unit dose patch. Dose delivered is determined by the site of application, the patch delivery rate and the surface area of the patch in contact with the skin [16, 17]. Louis [18] describes optimising buprenorphine dose by cutting the matrix style transdermal patch in half or quarter for individuals with chronic pain. Modifying TDDS requires careful consideration of the nature of the patch. This information for registered transdermal patches is typically presented in the approved product information. Cutting reservoir type patches significantly disrupts the integrity of the TDDS leading to excessive drug release and also occupational drug exposure to the healthcare professional.

Splitting Tablets

Tablet splitting is a common practice by patients and healthcare workers in aged care not only to aid in dose optimisation but also to reduce the cost of medicines [12]. The potential impact of tablet splitting needs to be carefully considered; from the patient perspective, it is essential to assess their physical (dexterity, strength, visual acuity) and cognitive ability to split tablets. A key factor is whether the tablet is scored to facilitate easy and accurate splitting. Marriot and Nation [12] highlighted that unusually shaped tablets can lead to inaccuracies in tablet splitting.

Quinzler et al. [19] investigated tablet splitting behaviour in the primary care setting in Germany using a cross-sectional questionnaire in 59 general practitioner practice sites involving 905 patients (taking 3,158 medicines). Overall, 24% of tablets were split and only 8.7% of all the split tablets were unscored, and 3.8% of all tablets split were not recommended to be split. Tablets of more expensive and higher strength medicines were twice as likely to be split. These authors also found that only 20% of the unscored tablet brands that were commonly split contained explicit information on dividing or splitting individual tablets and only 36.4% of the manufacturer's literature on the split brands that were not allowed to be split stated that splitting was inappropriate. The implication is that inappropriate splitting may have a significant clinical outcome.

A review by Noviasky et al. [20] evaluated the limited direct evidence of the safety and efficacy of split tablets in clinical trials. Split lisinopril tablets were as effective for hypertension as whole tablets of the same dose. Furthermore, split tablets of statins (such as atorvastatin, lovastatin and simvastatin) were no less effective as judged by cholesterol concentrations [20]. These authors also concluded, based on observational studies, that extended-release, enteric-coated or tablets that cannot be split accurately are inappropriate for splitting [20]. This and others work also observed that the accuracy of tablet splitting also depends on whether a device is used and on the skill of the user [21–23].

The following section discusses some of the strategies that can reduce the risks related to dose form modification.

Dose Form Modification: Some Guidelines

It is crucial that healthcare practitioners acknowledge that certain tablets or capsules are formulated in such a manner that they should only be swallowed whole and these medicines should not be crushed, broken or chewed. A comprehensive list of such products and information on them can be found in a number of resources (see Table 2). If such a case arises, alternative routes of administration or therapeutically equivalent medicines (with suitable dose forms) should be sought.

Once the impact of modification on safety and efficacy of medicine is established, then healthcare practitioners should ensure that they use suitable equipment and techniques for modifying the dose form including adequate staff protection. Dose form modification should be conducted using a glass mortar and pestle (or other non-porous equipment) that can be easily cleaned to minimise the risk of cross-patient contamination. For medicines that pose a significant risk to other patients or staff dedicated equipment should be used for each patient.

Table 2 Useful resources to establish the relative safety and risks associated with dose form modifications

Resource	Comment
Approved Product (API) and Consumer Medicines Information (CMI)	Every registered medicine has an API and CMI. These are an essential resource to inform the healthcare practitioners about the nature of the dose form and its optimal handling and storage conditions
Australia Medicines Handbook, *Drug Choice Companion (Age Care),* 2nd edition	Provides valuable insights into optimal and safe practices for dose form modification
Oral dosage forms that should not be crushed[a], Mitchell JF, Institute for Safe Medication Practices	A web resource (including many formulation and medicines available in North America) endorsed by the Institute for Safe Medication Practices
Do not crush list[b], Vincent M, Wollongong Hospital Pharmacy	A widely used and endorsed list that outlines the nature of each dose form and whether it is appropriate to modify this dose form
Guide to the handling of medication in nursing homes in NSW[c], NSW Health Department, Information Bulletin No. 2003/10 (2003)	Provides valuable insights into optimal and safe practices for dose form modification
Guidelines for medication management in residential aged care facilities[d], Australian Pharmaceutical Advisory Council, 2002, 3rd edition	Provides valuable insights into optimal and safe practices for dose form modification
Consensus guideline on the medication management of adults with swallowing difficulties, Wright D, Chapman N, Foundling-Miah M, Greenwall R, Griffith R, Guyon A, Merriman H	Excellent check for decision making in patients with difficulty swallowing

[a] http://www.ismp.org/tools/donotcrush.pdf (accessed 24 Sept 2008)
[b] http://www.health.nsw.gov.au/quality/natmed/pdf/DoNotCrushListSample.pdf (accessed 24 Sept 2008)
[c] http://www.health.nsw.gov.au/policies/PD/2005/pdf/PD2005_105.pdf (accessed 24 Sept 2008)
[d] http://www.health.gov.au/internet/main/publishing.nsf/Content/nmp-publications-apac.htm (accessed 24 Sept 2008)

It is possible that generally multiple tablets may be crushed together but some medicines should not be combined (Table 2). When capsule and tablets are to be administered together, it is appropriate to crush the tablets first and then open the capsules and add the powder or pellets (without further crushing) contained therein to the crushed tablets. Once crushed, tablets may be mixed with a small amount of a soft food to facilitate administration. However, some drugs should not be mixed or taken with dairy products (e.g. yoghurt). The modified dose forms should be administered immediately unless there is relevant data to confirm their physiochemical stability. Patients should remain upright (where possible) when medication is administered and adequate fluid should be administered to facilitate oesophageal transit. Details of the modification and administration procedure of the medicines should be recorded on the medication chart or clinical notes. Patients should be routinely monitored to establish the appropriate therapeutic response to all medications, especially those that have been administered in a modified form.

Conclusion

Dose form modification is an increasingly common practice in the age care setting where it can facilitate drug administration; however, it also carries the risk of medication inefficacy, enhanced risk of excessive therapeutic effects or occupational exposure to potentially harmful medicines for healthcare practitioners. Practices, such as tablet crushing and capsule opening, require careful attention to issues such as formulation characteristics, drug stability, medicine palatability and physiochemical interactions. Healthcare practitioners should consult pharmacists to ensure that pharmaceutical and clinical implications of dose form modification receive due consideration.

References

1. Hilmer SN, McLachlan A, Le Couteur DG (2007) Clinical pharmacology in geriatric patients. Fundam Clin Pharmacol 21:217–230
2. Australian Pharmaceutical Advisory Council (2006) Guiding principles for medication management in the community. http://www.health.gov.au/internet/main/publishing.nsf/Content/nmp-publications-apac.htm. Accessed 24 Sept 2008
3. Australian Pharmaceutical Advisory Council (2002) Guidelines for medication management in residential aged care facilities, 3rd edn. Australian Pharmaceutical Advisory Council, Canberra, November 2002. http://www.health.gov.au/internet/main/publishing.nsf/Content/nmp-publications-apac.htm. Accessed 24 Sept 2008
4. Stubbs J, Haw C, Dickens G (2008) Dose form modification – a common but potentially hazardous practice. A literature review and study of medication administration to older psychiatric inpatients. Int Psychogeriatr 20:616–627
5. NSW Health Department (2003) Guide to the handling of medication in nursing homes in NSW. Information Bulletin No 2003/10, NSW Health Department, North Sydney, 27 May 2003. http://www.agpn.com.au/client_images/23110.pdf. Accessed 24 Sept 2008

6. Morris H (2006) Dysphagia in the elderly – a management challenge for nurses. Br J Nurs 15:558–562
7. Carnaby-Mann G, Crary M (2005) Pill swallowing by adults with dysphagia. Arch Otolaryngol Head Neck Surg 131:970–975
8. Wright D (2002) Medication administration in nursing homes. Nurs Stand 16:33–38
9. Hanssens Y, Woods D, Alsulaiti A, Adheir F, Al-Meer N, Obaidan N (2006) Improving oral medicine administration in patients with swallowing problems and feeding tubes. Ann Pharmacother 40:2142–2147
10. van den Bemt PM, Cusell MB, Overbeeke PW, Trommelen M, van Dooren D, Ophorst WR, Egberts AC (2006) Quality improvement of oral medication administration in patients with enteral feeding tubes. Qual Saf Health Care 15:44–47
11. Haw C, Stubbs J, Dickens G (2007) An observational study of medication administration errors in old-age psychiatric inpatients. Int J Qual Health Care 19:210–216
12. Marriott J, Nation R (2002) Splitting tablets. Aust Prescr 25:133–135
13. Cleary JD, Evans PC, Hikal AH, Chapman SW (1999) Administration of crushed extended-release pentoxifylline tablets: bioavailability and adverse effects. Am J Health Syst Pharm 56:1529–1534
14. Jordan S, Griffiths H, Griffith R (2003) Administration of medicines, part 2: pharmacology. Nurs Stand 18:45–54
15. Kirkevold Ø, Engedal K (2005) Concealment of drugs in food and beverages in nursing homes: cross-sectional study. BMJ 330:20–22
16. Kaestli LZ, Wasilewski-Rasca AF, Bonnabry P, Vogt-Ferrier N (2008) Use of transdermal drug formulations in the elderly. Drugs Aging 25:269–280
17. Ranade VV (1991) Drug delivery systems. 6. Transdermal drug delivery. J Clin Pharmacol 31:401–18
18. Louis F (2006) Transdermal buprenorphine in pain management – experiences from clinical practice: five case studies. Int J Clin Pract 60:1330–1334
19. Quinzler R, Gasse C, Schneider A, Kaufmann-Kolle P, Szecsenyi J, Haefeli WE (2006) The frequency of inappropriate tablet splitting in primary care. Eur J Clin Pharmacol 62:1065–1073
20. Noviasky J, Lo V, Luft DD, Saseen J (2006) Clinical inquiries. Which medications can be split without compromising efficacy and safety? J Fam Pract 55:707–708
21. Quinzler R, Szecsenyi J, Haefeli WE (2007) Tablet splitting: patients and physicians need better support. Eur J Clin Pharmacol 63:1203–1204
22. Peek BT, Al-Achi A, Coombs SJ (2002) Accuracy of tablet splitting by elderly patients. JAMA 288:451–452
23. Mitchell JE (2000) Oral dosage forms that should not be crushed: 2000 update. Hosp Pharm 35:553–557

Electronic Health Records, Medications, and Long-Term Care

F. Michael Gloth

Keywords Electronic health records • Electronic medical records • Personal health records • Information technology

What is EHR?

An electronic health record (EHR) can be defined as a comprehensive computerized record system that contains the medical record, results of labs, imaging, and other tests, consultant information, prescribing information, and oftentimes incorporates computerized order entry as well as other features, which may involve billing, prior authorization, assessment of drug–drug interactions, decision support mechanisms, and more.

Other terms, such as personal health record (PHR) and electronic medical record (EMR), have also been used almost interchangeably, but they do have slightly different definitions. Usually an EMR is more limited than an EHR, and a PHR may have an abundance of other information, which an individual patient elects to accrue regardless of its relevance to the physician or the healthcare provider overseeing a person's medical care.

In a PHR, a person may elect to collect all of his or her daily finger stick information from home, articles on health tips or diseases that he or she deems important, etc. For the sole purpose of simplicity, this chapter will deal exclusively with EHRs.

How Can an EHR Affect Medication Management?

An Institute of Medicine report released in 2000 increased awareness about patient care as it relates to medical errors [1]. The proposals to resolve the problem were very predictable and ranged from increased regulation to public reporting of information

F.M. Gloth (✉)
Division of Geriatric Medicine and Gerontology, Johns Hopkins University School of Medicine, Baltimore, MD, USA
e-mail: fgloth1@jhmi.edu

S. Koch et al. (eds.), *Medication Management in Older Adults:*
A Concise Guide for Clinicians, DOI 10.1007/978-1-60327-457-9_9,
© Springer Science+Business Media, LLC 2010

(e.g., Nursing home reports from the Minimum Data Set (MDS), Joint Commission on the Accreditation of Healthcare Organizations (JCAHO)), survey scores, or various state survey results, which have historically been costly and burdensome in their distraction from patient care, in addition to the fact that they have lacked adequate data to link them to improved outcomes.

One solution that has received a favorable review from physicians and patients alike is the use of EHRs [2]. In addition to the opportunities offered by computerized order entry (see chapter "Computerized Order Entry," on this topic), which may be part of an EHR system, there are many other merits that argue for obtaining an EHR as a means of reducing medication errors.

Despite such potential, EHR has not been as widely embraced by physicians as has been seen in other consumer-based environments. Charles Safran from Harvard Medical School noted, "The promise of electronic patient record is real and proven, but the reality for physicians in the United States has been largely unrealized" [3]. This was recently reiterated in an article from the *New England Journal of Medicine*, showing that less than 20% of physicians in the USA were using a comprehensive EHR system for patient records [4].

Consider the many opportunities for improved medication management with EHR. Such systems eliminated transcriptions errors associated with the deciphering of illegible handwriting. By providing electronic prescriptions directly to the pharmacy, another opportunity for transcription errors or misunderstood verbal communications can be obviated. Such systems can also improve the efficiency of medical note writing and various aspects of medical information gathering and dissemination [5].

By contributing to improved access of information, the duplication of medications or classes of medications can be minimized. Such can be the result of improved quality assurance as data is more readily available for review of practice patterns and outcomes (even when the reviewer is offsite!), or with the elimination of obstacles created by lost, misplaced, or inaccessible medical charts. Simply knowing what has been ordered previously can reduce redundant testing and prescription writing.

Having almost instant access to information, increases the time available to provide clinical care and review medications. Communication among various providers can also lend to opportunities for improved coordination of care.

Decision support found with some EHR systems also can provide clinicians with information on appropriate medication selection, dosing, and frequency. EHR systems that provide medication adjudication programs can identify inappropriate drugs and potential drug–drug interactions as well. Some EHR systems provide an option for online access to medical information websites while in the patient record. This allows for review of medications, while the patient is still in the office and, thus, counseling can take place while the patient is onsite. Such options also allow for patient education materials to be accessed and either printed before the patient's departure or to be shared with the patient for additional access after the patient leaves the office.

Opportunities from EHR also include the ability to provide decision support that is based on diagnosis, institutional guidelines, formulary options, and treatment recommendations from nationally recognized resources. Depending on the flexibility of systems, they can even adjust relatively quickly to alterations in prescribing recommendations based on recent research and changes in standards for medical care.

Additionally, EHR can facilitate changes in prescribing behavior as well as other practices in medicine. For example, an EHR, which included advance directives in the history and physical format, led to the documentation of advance directive conversations in almost all patients within the first month of its use [6]. Given the difficulty in changing behaviors of physicians, the EHR has great promise for providing improvement in prescriber practice patterns with relatively little effort.

EHR also may offer options for calculating or taking into account parameters that may affect prescribing. For example, body mass index (BMI), renal function, and age could all be calculated on a patient based on the EHR data gathered. Subsequently, adjustments or recommendations for them can be made in real time. This should help to improve efficacy as well as reduce adverse events.

Patient/Caregiver Involvement Through EHR Can Improve Care

EHR offers improvement in another form of communication. Patients and family members, who have authorization, can potentially review information from recent patient interactions with the healthcare system and make inquiries electronically in a secure fashion. Recently, it has been demonstrated that an accessible EHR can improve medication reconciliation with the assistance of patients and family members who can review medications online [7].

Patients and or their caregivers who find discrepancies between medications on the electronic medication list and either the types of medication or the dosing of medications can contact their healthcare provider and remedy the conflict. Presumably, this can be done with two potential benefits. Either the patient can start to take the medication as prescribed or the practitioner will learn that the way that patient is actually taking the medication has been more beneficial and can modify the medication list to reflect the actual dose, medication, or both.

Technology also exists for relevant clinical information to be obtained at home and electronically submitted to the EHR database. For example, blood pressure readings in hypertensives or glucose monitoring in diabetics can be transmitted electronically to a clinician via the internet or phone system, and this information can be downloaded directly into the EHR.

EHR Still May Have Some Drawbacks for Medication Management

While the discussion thus far may be compelling and clearly in support of using EHR, the reader should not assume that EHR is problem free. There are potential errors inherent when using EHR.

Most obvious is the ability to reproduce erroneous information on a far larger scale than with paper charts. Allergy documentation or incorrect medication entry can be propagated to every provider in seconds.

EHR systems that are too cumbersome or that overload the clinician with information run the risk of being avoided or ignored. For example, if every time a clinician orders a medication, a drug–drug interaction, or a warning shows up that is either irrelevant or sufficiently minor as to simply be a distraction, clinicians will start to ignore the warning screens or even turn of the feature, if the option to do so exists.

Systems also must be secure. Systems will not be used, if the patient or clinician is not confident that the medical information or the prescribing techniques are anything less that private and secure.

Another potential problem that has rarely been articulated has to do with interoperability and interface development. What this means is that a program that has an interface to be able to assimilate information from another program with either a similar language or even a completely different coding background infrastructure. When such interfaces are developed, testing should take place to be sure that the information into the system is reflected by what the EHR system puts out. In essence, when laboratory information developed using a background language called SNOMED is received by an EHR working with an HL-7 infrastructure, what is recognized as hemoglobin of 12 g/dL in SNOMED, is also featured as hemoglobin of 12 g/dL in the HL-7-based EHR. Where potential problems may arise is when upgrades are performed for different products independently. If an upgrade at either end results in a change that affects the interface, there is a risk that data will not be properly assimilated any longer. In such an instance, incorrect information could be transmitted without anyone knowing it. Conceivably, this could happen on a relatively large scale unless proper testing was performed in advance to assure that such operations remain consistent and accurate between systems.

Conclusion

EHR offers a unique opportunity to improve medication management through increased efficiency and removal of adverse events associated with traditional prescribing methods. Eliminating illegible handwriting, copying errors, and duplicate prescriptions are all direct examples of how EHR systems can assist with medication management.

Improving patient compliance with access to medication information online also is a potential benefit to EHR. Physician support for decision making and medication selection and dosing are also opportunities for improved medication management fostered by EHR. Other advantages are outlined in Table 1.

Table 1 Areas where EHR can help with medication management

(1) Eliminate illegibility
(2) Reduce transcription errors
(3) Facilitate data collection and analysis for quality improvement
(4) Allow for real-time decision support, including medication selection
(5) Improve continuity by increasing the availability of information across the continuum of care, including current medication instructions, prior prescriptions, and testing
(6) Provide access to important clinical information, for example, weights, creatinine clearance, potential drug–drug interactions, etc.
(7) Provide prompts and screening or monitoring tools for clinicians

While EHR has great promise in augmenting medication management, it does not come without the need for caution related to security and the potential for different types of medication errors that can suddenly be propagated on a very large scale. With appropriate precautions and the development of appropriate standards, however, EHR is likely to change the way medications are managed, especially for older adults. This will mean fewer medication errors and early detection of those that do occur.

References

1. Kohn LT, Corrigan JM, Donaldson MS (eds) (2000) To err is human: building a safer health system. Committee on quality of health care in American Institute of Medicine. National Academy, Washington
2. Rundle RL (2002) Healthcare providers let patients view records online. Wall Street J, p B1
3. Safran C (2001) Electronic medical records: a decade of experience. JAMA 285:1766
4. DesRoches CM, Campbell EG, Rao SR et al (2008) Electronic health records in ambulatory care – a national survey of physicians. N Engl J Med 359:50–60
5. Safran C, Rind DM, Davis RB et al (1995) Guidelines for the management of HIV infection in a computer-based medical record. Lancet 246:341–346
6. Personal communication from Victory Springs Senior Health Associates on instituting Smart E-Records
7. Siteman E, Businger A, Gandhi T, Grant R, Poon E, Schnipper J, Volk L, Wald J, Middleton B (2007) Physicians value patient review of their electronic health record data as a means to improve accuracy of medication list documentation. AMIA Annu Symp Proc 11:1116

Computerized Order Entry

F. Michael Gloth

Keywords Computerized order entry • Physician order entry • Electronic prescribing • Health information technology

Potential to Reduce Medication Errors

As this book attests, there are many reasons for individuals to experience medical errors and adverse events. Oftentimes, medication problems are precipitated through a cascade of events. In the ideal setting, a clinician prescriber identifies an appropriate medication, writes an appropriate prescription, the prescription is transported to the pharmacist or relayed by some other mechanism to the pharmacist, the prescription is filled, delivered, and after being dispensed in the appropriate quantity, it is administered as prescribed. Errors at any point along the chain can lead to errors and adverse events. In every place wherein an individual has the opportunity to alter a prescription, there is an opportunity to create a medication error. Thus, any process that reduces transcribing or otherwise manually relaying medication information is an opportunity to reduce medication error.

To this end, e-prescribing or computerized order entry (COE) (also sometimes called electronic physician order entry or computerized physician order entry) has created an environment with great potential to reduce medication errors.

What is COE?

COE, sometimes called computerized prescriber order entry (CPOE) involves electronically entering information at some point along the chain from the point of prescription to the point of dispersing and administering the medication and recording

F.M. Gloth (✉)
Division of Geriatric Medicine and Gerontology, Johns Hopkins University School of Medicine, Baltimore, MD, USA
e-mail: fgloth1@jhmi.edu

S. Koch et al. (eds.), *Medication Management in Older Adults:*
A Concise Guide for Clinicians, DOI 10.1007/978-1-60327-457-9_10,
© Springer Science+Business Media, LLC 2010

that action. In the best of worlds, the physician or other healthcare provider enters the information in a computerized format. Any adverse interactions or other problems are determined at that point and the clinician is given electronic guidance regarding the potential problem. The physician enters the finalized prescription, which is electronically transferred directly to the pharmacist with copies being sent to other personnel capable of delivering the end product.

In a completely automated environment, medication dosage and quantity are dispensed at the pharmacy level or at the point of administration depending on the sophistication of technology in place. There is a review of the medication at the level of the pharmacy and at the point of administration in many institutionalized settings. This may involve a confirmatory process with a patient identifier, such as a wrist band. Such patient identifiers may simply be visual, for example, printed names, or more technologically advanced information, for example, a barcode. Where barcodes are used, the barcode on the prescription must match that on the patient and, after confirmation, medication is administered.

Advantages of COE

COE minimizes the likelihood that an individual will get the wrong medication, the wrong dose, or the wrong administration time. Common errors in legibility with written prescriptions, errors in transcribing from one form to another, along with other common human errors are virtually eliminated.

Such an order entry also has been demonstrated to be more cost-effective with fewer medication duplications, fewer drug interactions, and greater ease with formulary adherence [1, 2]. Table 1 outlines reasons to expect improved medication management with COE.

Table 1 Potential advantages to computerized order entry

Potential COE advantages
Improved legibility
More rapid communication to and from pharmacy
Less opportunity for drug diversion
Greater access for other authorized healthcare providers (especially with an EHR)
Can be integrated into decision-support systems
Electronic link to drug–drug interaction warnings
Can access prescribing physician
Can access prescribing history
Can more readily access allergies and adverse drug reaction history
Additional information can be obtained in real time while seeing the patient
Patient education materials can be generated at point of contact
Quality assurance is more efficient with opportunity for immediate data analysis, including postmarketing reporting
Potentially less costly
Nonpunitive formulary guidance

Potential Pitfalls with COE

While electronic prescribing may minimize opportunities for drug diversion, reduce errors associated with illegibility, and foster a more streamlined approach, there remain opportunities for medication errors even with electronic prescribing [3]. While errors in software programming can occur, these are exceedingly rare. More commonly errors at the level of order entry can occur and be propagated at the relatively large scale.

With COE, there may no longer be an issue in distinguishing between whether a medication is ordered in milligrams or micrograms once entered, however, should such an error occur in the original prescription, it is conceivable that the wrong dose of the medication could be given for a relatively long period of time. Subsequently, such a replicated error could lead to toxicity. Alternatively, a large number of erroneous prescriptions could be distributed inappropriately *en mass*. For example, should a prescriber inadvertently order a vaccine for chicken pox as opposed to the vaccine for shingles commonly administered to people over the age of 60, it is conceivable that a large cohort of individuals would get the wrong medication and this would be propagated due to the duplicative capacity of electronic prescribing.

Other problems have developed where adjustments in medications have been made without using electronic entry when such access exists. A prescription written in the traditional manner may not be transformed into the electronic system. A system that does not have the ability to recognize such changes may make it difficult to administer the newly prescribed dose without first having the old dose electronically canceled and another electronic prescription written.

In systems where changes are not easily made in an existing prescription with COE, it is possible to have multiple orders for the same drug. Systems that require cancelation of an old order and entry of a new one for the same drug of different dosing or scheduling otherwise may offer the potential for duplication and, therefore, toxicity or other adverse events. Ideally, COE will allow for adjustment of medication dosing and electronically, and, in an automated fashion, cancel and record the old prescription, while updating to the new dose and frequency. This helps to avoid the danger that a patient could get both the old dose that was prescribed concomitantly with the new dose.

Drug-to-Drug Interactions and Information Overload

COE can also provide electronic monitoring for potential drug–drug interactions. While this has great potential to reduce such interactions, there is a danger in overloading the clinician with excessive and pedantic information. Should the prescriber feel that the information is redundant and/or excessively cautious without a mechanism to switch repeat reminders off, then there is the chance that the prescriber will ignore or dismiss all warnings, making the monitoring system ineffective. Many such systems come as an add-on to COE systems and the cost for these additional services may be prohibitively expensive.

Selecting the Right COE

Like EHR systems, there are a host of COE systems from which to choose. A solo or small office practice may find that the needs vary considerably from those of a large health system. The environment may require greater or lesser complexity depending upon the make-up of the practice settings.

Most systems have a few basic features, which most providers will need. However, there is tremendous variation, and the selection of a system is based on the variability of vendors and the systems being sold. Instead of changing your system to fit the COE System, try to find a system that fits yours.

A COE system should allow prescribers to enter and manage multiple order types quickly and securely, both onsite, as well as, offsite, at any time. The system should be accessible in a role-specific fashion to any provider who can and should facilitate the process. This means pharmacists, nurse practitioners, physician assistants, nurses, and laboratory, radiology, and other medical technologists, as well as the physician.

Ideally, the system should integrate with the necessary pharmacy systems as well as the EHR being used by the practitioner. It is usually desirable to have selected patient- and drug-specific information available to the prescribers at the time of ordering.

Some systems are stock off-the-shelf systems with little option for modification. The best systems allow some features to be customized to accommodate prescriber preferences, protocols, etc. Ideally, unwanted features can be silenced or placed in the background as well.

The COE system chosen should not only communicate directly with the pharmacy or an electronic prescription vendor that communicates with multiple pharmacies, but it should also be able to produce hard copy prescriptions and fax information for situations, when the usual pharmacy is not the patient's pharmacy of choice.

The COE or electronic health record (EHR) working in concert with the COE should be able to incorporate demographic and clinical information so that minimal additional information needs to be entered when providing prescriptions, new orders, or discharge instructions. The COE should also be accessible for federally mandated medication reconciliation.

As mentioned earlier, one feature that is useful in reducing duplicative orders is to have a COE system that allows the prescriber to electronically change the order type without having to reenter the order or D/C, the prior order. With minimal effort on the computer, the prescriber should also be able to change an order from one setting to another without rewriting each order. For example, one should be able to go from an inpatient order to an ambulatory care order and vice versa.

Administrative Features

Prescribing recommendations and upgrades will happen. The health system or prescriber should be able to update recommendations and prescribing protocols easily while working within the patient record and not have to go to a separate set of templates after closing out of the patient record.

Likewise, the health system or office should not have to upgrade its existing computer hardware to support the COE software selected. Ideally, the product will be web-based with upgrades occurring without disruption of patient care and without additional resource utilization from the healthcare system or office.

Depending upon the work environment, a COE compatible with a personal digital assistant (PDA) may be preferred. Such consideration of current practices will go a long way in fostering buy-in from staff.

Security and Standards

Security features will be of paramount importance. The COE must provide levels of data encryption that would comply with Health Insurance Portability and Accountability Act (HIPAA) requirements. New standards are being developed for EHR and COE at a national level. The prudent buyer will take this into account and inquire what accommodations a vendor will make should standards be developed that turn out to be different from what the COE currently accommodates.

Overall, there should be adequate interoperability in any system selected so that communication with other providers, vendors, labs, etc. will be seamless and quick. The ancillary healthcare providers employed to assist prescribers should be accommodated in a fashion that enables identification of the ancillary providers with role-specific authorization in conjunction with the prescriber. This may allow prescribers to simply review and then finalize the process with a single sign-off.

Whatever is selected must provide regulatory compliance and facilitate that process throughout the prescribing practice. There should also be sufficient built-in flexibility to handle regulatory changes down the road, as best as one can predict.

Training and Portability

Always understand what training a vendor is willing to provide, what level of support will be available after a system is purchased and how updates are handled. An additional consideration is the accessibility to patients and caregivers who are authorized to review such information. Ask whether there is access for patients and authorized family or caregivers offsite and whether such information is portable should they move or otherwise go outside of the system for health care.

Conclusion

COE has the potential to reduce medication errors typically seen with handwritten prescription processes. Improved legibility, efficiency, information access, and reduced human contact provide many opportunities to improve medication management in older adults.

The technological advantages can be offset to some degree by new categories of potential medication error propagated by the new format. Deciding upon the right COE system that complements the environment in which it will be used is important in optimizing medication management. Table 2 gives some features to consider when selecting COE systems.

Table 2 Selection criteria for computerized order entry systems

Basic COE features
- Find the COE system that fits you rather than you changing to fit the COE system
- Entry of multiple order types should be quick
- Entry must be secure and HIPAA compliant
- Access should be available anytime, anywhere
- Access should be role-specific for any provider with a direct clinical care role
- It should have adequate interoperability
- It should provide selected patient- and drug-specific information to the prescribers at the time of ordering
- There should be sufficient malleable to accommodate prescriber preferences, protocols, etc. Ideally, unwanted features can be silenced or placed in the background as well
- The COE system should be flexible enough to produce hard copy prescriptions and FAX information for situations, when the usual pharmacy is not the patients pharmacy of choice
- The COE should be able to download demographic and clinical information so that minimal additional information needs to be entered when providing prescriptions, new orders, or discharge instructions
- Medication reconciliation should be a feature
- Allows the prescriber to electronically change the order type without having to reenter the order or DC, the prior order
- Able to change an order from one setting to another without rewriting each order

Administrative features
- Able to update recommendations and prescribing protocols easily while working within the patient record
- Web-based with upgrades occurring without disruption of patient care and without additional resource utilization from the healthcare system or office
- Compatible with current practice, e.g., personal digital assistant (PDA)

Security and standards
- Provides levels of data encryption that would comply with Health Insurance Portability and Accountability Act (HIPAA) requirements.
- Takes development of new standards into account
- Interoperability with other providers, vendors, labs, etc. seamless and quick.
- Accommodates ancillary providers with role-specific authorization in conjunction with the prescriber
- Provides regulatory compliance and built-in flexibility to handle regulatory changes down the road, as best as one can predict

Training and portability
- Support available after a system is purchased
- Easy and inexpensive update process
- Accessibility to patients and authorized caregivers
- Portable

When the correct system is in place and used correctly, one can expect far superior medication management, particularly for an older more vulnerable population of adults.

References

1. Brown SH, Lincoln MJ, Groen PJ, Kolodner RM (2003) VistA – U.S. Department of Veterans Affairs national-scale HIS. Int J Med Inform 69:135–156. Online access http://www1.va.gov/cprsdemo/docs/VistA_Int_Jrnl_Article.pdf Accessed 9 Jan 2008
2. Bates DW, Leape LL, Cullen DJ et al (1998) Effect of computerized physician order entry and a team intervention on prevention of serious medication errors. JAMA 280:1311–1316
3. Koppel R, Metlay JP, Cohen A et al (2005) Role of computerized physician order entry systems in facilitating medication errors. JAMA 293:1197–1203

Inappropriate Prescribing: Beers Criteria, Polypharmacy, and Drug Burden

F. Michael Gloth

Keywords Inappropriate medication use • Older adults • Geriatrics • Beers criteria • Polypharmacy • Adverse drug events • Adverse drug reactions

Beers Criteria

In 2003, an article entitled, "Updating the Beers Criteria for Potentially Inappropriate Medication Use in Older Adults" was published in the Archives of Internal Medicine (Fick et al. [1]). This article summarized the results of the consensus panel of experts from various disciplines (see Table 1), who had a wealth of experience dealing with seniors and had extensively evaluated the literature on adverse events in older adults.

The updated report was based on a modified Delphi method for formulating group judgment and the assessment on such data. On the basis of this evaluation, the group reported on medications or medication classes that should generally be avoided in seniors (persons aged above 65 years), either because such medications were ineffective or they posed an unnecessarily high risk with safer alternatives being available. Additionally, they addressed medications that should not be used in older persons who have specific medical conditions. This report was a reevaluation of the criteria that had been reviewed earlier (in 1997) as well as an update on new conditions or considerations that had not been addressed in that earlier report.

Method of Evaluation

The modified Delphi method employed solicitation from individuals for responses to a survey. A review of responses includes an evaluation for variance and the means to determine the questions for which the group has reached a

F.M. Gloth (✉)
Division of Geriatric Medicine and Gerontology, Johns Hopkins University School of Medicine, Baltimore, MD, USA
e-mail: fgloth1@jhmi.edu

S. Koch et al. (eds.), *Medication Management in Older Adults:*
A Concise Guide for Clinicians, DOI 10.1007/978-1-60327-457-9_11,
© Springer Science+Business Media, LLC 2010

Table 1 Updated Beers criteria U.S. consensus panel of experts

Mark H. Beers M.D	Merck & Co. Inc., West Point, PA
Maude Babington, PharmD	Babington Consulting LLC, Boulder, CO
Manju T. Beier, PharmD	University of Michigan, Ann Arbor
Richard W. Besdine, MD	Brown University Providence, Rhode Island
Jack Fincham, PhD	University of Kansas, Lawrence
F. Michael Gloth, III, MD	Johns Hopkins University School of Medicine, Baltimore, MD
Thomas Jackson MD	Medical College of Georgia, Augusta
John E. Morley, MD	St. Louis University Health Sciences Center, St. Louis, MO
Beck Neagle, PharmD, BCPC	Medco Health Solutions, Franklin Lakes, NJ
Todd Semla, Pharm D, MS	Evanston Northwestern Health Care, Evanston, IL
Mark A. Stratin, PharmD	University of Oklahoma City
Andrew D. Weinberg, MD	Emery University School of Medicine Atlanta, GA
Donna M. Fick, PhD, RN	Department of Veterans Affairs, Medical Center, Augusta
James W. Cooper PhD, RPH	Department of Clinical and Administrative Pharmacy College of Pharmacy, University of Georgia, Athens
William E. Wade, PharmD	Department of Clinical and Administrative Pharmacy College of Pharmacy, University of Georgia, Athens
Jennifer L. Waller, PhD	Office of Biostatistics Medical College of Georgia, Augusta
Ross MacLean, MD	Department of Medicine Center for Healthcare Improvement Medical College of Georgia, Augusta

consensus. Additionally, there was an extensive literature review incorporating articles published from January 1994 to the present time. The articles reviewed were in English and described or analyzed medications used by (ambulatory) seniors living in the community living (ambulatory) seniors, and those living in nursing homes.

On the basis of that literature review, a table and bibliography was created. Medline was used for searching items with key terms "adverse drug reactions, adverse drug events, medication problems, and medications and elderly." Additionally, there was a hand search and identification of additional references based on bibliographies of relevant articles, and finally all panelists were invited to add references and articles. Every study was systematically reviewed by two investigators with particular focus on study design, sample size, medications reviewed, summary of results and key points, quality type and category of medications addressed in the severity of drug-related problems.

Selection of Panelists

Panelist had been selected based on experience and judgment including extensive clinical practice, publications in the area, and/or senior academic rank. They were also chosen to represent acute, long-term, and community practice settings with pharmacological, geriatric medicine, and psychiatric expertise.

Medication Selection

Based on this in-depth review, a table was created of 48 individual medications or classes of medications that should probably be avoided in older adults along with the potential concerns. A second table was created listing 20 diseases or conditions and medications that should not be given to seniors having such conditions.

Classes of drugs that are recommended not to be used in older adults overall include:

- *Muscle relaxants and antispasmodics,* because of the poor tolerability in older adults related to anticholinergic activities, sedation, and weakness;
- *Gastrointestinal antispasmodic drugs,* due to their highly anticholinergic activity and uncertain effectiveness;
- *Anticholinergics and antihistamines* overall (both nonprescription as well as prescription), since many of these have potent anticholinergic properties (nonanticholinergic antihistamines are preferred in older adults in treating allergic reactions);
- *Ergot mesyloids (Hydergine) and cyclandelate*, because of the insufficient data to show effectiveness in the doses studied;
- Any *ferrysulfate product containing more than 325 mg* or dosing beyond 325 mg in a day, because these do not dramatically increase the amount absorbed but greatly increase the incidence of constipation;
- All *barbiturates* with the exception of Phenobarbital, since they are felt to be inappropriate except when used to control seizures due to the highly addictive nature of these drugs and the likelihood that they will cause more adverse effects;
- And most *sedative or hypnotic drugs* in older adults. Some drugs have been identified through the Beers panel as having greater severity than others.

A distinction among drugs has been classified by the Beers panel as either a severity rating of "high" or "low." Those drugs identified under the "high" severity rating can be seen in Table 2).

Other drugs on the list with lower severity ratings include: propoxyphene (Darvon in combinations therefore), digoxin (Lanoxin not to exceed 0.125 mg per day except when treating atrial arrhythmias), short acting dipyridamole (Persantine), reserpine at doses greater than 0.25 mg, Hydergine, cyclandelate (Cyclospasmol), fera sulfate greater than 325 mg per day, cyclandelate (Cyclospasmol), isoxsuprine (Vasodilan), doxazosin (Cardura), clonidine (Catapres), cimetidine (Tagamet), methacrylic acid (Edecrin), and estrogens (oral).

Reasoning for Categorization

The reason for the selection of the drugs listed above are varied but all are identified as agents that place older adults in unnecessary risk for adverse events either independently or in comparison to other safer agents with equivalent efficacy. Propoxyphene is an example of an agent that offers few analgesic advantages over even acetaminophen; yet, it has adverse effects of other narcotic agents. For people

Table 2 High-risk drugs from revised Beers criteria

Alprazolam (Xanax greater than 2 mg)
Amiodarone (Cordarone)
Amitriptyline (Elavil) and amitriptyline-containing drugs
Belladonna alkaloids (Donnatal, etc.)
Carisoprodol (Soma)
Chlorazepate (Tranxene)
Chlordiazepoxide (Librium) and chlordiazepoxide-containing drugs
Chlorpheniramine (chlor-Trimeton)
Chlorpropamide (Diabinese)
Chlorzoxazone (Paraflex)
Cyclobenzaprine (Flexeril)
Cyproheptadine (Periactin)
Desiccated thyroid
Dexchlorpheniramine (Polaramine)
Diazepam (vallum)
Dicyclomine (Bentyl)
Diphenhydramine (Benadryl)
Disopyramide (Norpace, Norpace CR)
Doxepin (Sinequan)
Fluoxetine (Prozac) daily
Flurazepam (Dalmane)
Guanadrel (Hylorel)
Guanethidine (Ismelin)
Halazepam (Pexipam)
Hydroxyzine (Vistaril, Atarax)
Hyoscyamine (Levsin, Levsinex)
Indomethacin (Indocin, Indocin SR)
Ketolac (Toradol)
Lorazepam (Ativan greater than 3 mg)
Meperidine (Demerol)
Meprobamate (Miltown, Equanil)
Mesoridazine (Serentil)
Metaxalone (Skelaxin)
Methocarbamol (Robaxin)
Methyldopa (Aldomet) and methyldopa-containing drugs
Methyltestosterone (Android, Virilon, and Testred)
Mineral oil
Nifedipine (short acting Procardia and Adalat)
Nitrofurantoin (Macrodantin)
Orphenadrine (Norflex)
Oxazepam (Serax greater than 60 mg)
Oxybutynin (Ditropan, exclusive of Ditropan XL)
Pentazocine (Talwin)
Promethazine (Phenergan)
Propantheline (pro-Banthine)
Quazepam (Doral)

(continued)

Table 2 (continued)

Temazepam (Restoril greater than 15 mg)
Thioridazine (Mellaril)
Ticlopidine (Ticlid)
Triazolam (Halcion greater than 0.25 mg)
Trimethobenzamide (Tigan)
Tripelennamine

who have taken propoxyphene for long periods without adverse effects and found the drug to be an effective analgesic, it may not be necessary to discontinue the agent in place of another analgesic, but, certainly, individuals who are not successfully being treated with propoxyphene should not be given this as a first-line agent. Rather, alternatives, such as acetaminophen and other nonopioids, should be considered initially.

All nonsteroidal inflammatory drugs (NSAIDs) can be considered relatively dangerous in older adults for prolonged periods of time. Indomethacin produces the most CNS adverse events and therefore is discouraged in particular for use in older adults. The American Geriatrics Society is updated its guidelines on the management of persistent pain in older adults and NSAIDs receive additional scrutiny. Trimethobenzamide is one of the least effective antiemetic drugs but can cause extrapyramidal adverse effects. Amitriptyline is a commonly prescribed antidepressant both to treat depression as well as being used occasionally for neuropathic pain intervention. Because of the strong anticholinergic and sedation properties which contribute to a high risk of falls among other adverse events, amitriptyline should be avoided in an older adult population. Anticholinergic and sedating properties of doxepin also make this a drug to be avoided for seniors.

Disopyramide is the most potent negative anatrope of all antiarrhythmic drugs and therefore should be avoided due to the likelihood of inducing heart failure in older adults. It is also strongly anticholinergic and hence other antiarrhythmics should be selected. Digoxin is listed because of its decreased renal clearance in older adults, which may lead to increased risk of toxic events. Short-acting dipyridamole can cause orthostatic hypotension.

Chlorpropamide can induce depression, sedation and orthostatic hypotension and has a prolonged half-life in older adults, which can lead to prolonged hypoglycemia; additionally, it is the only oral hypoglycemic agent that causes SIADH. Diphenhydramine is often used as an agent for sleep. This agent, however, is likely to cause confusion and risk of falls and generally should be avoided. Even when used to treat allergic reactions, it should be used in the smallest possible dose.

Meperidine is generally not an effective oral analgesic in doses commonly used but it commonly causes confusion and has many disadvantages to the other narcotic drugs including an increased risk of falls relative to other opioids and a tendency to decrease seizure threshold. Ticlopidine may be more toxic than aspirin, and safer, more effective alternatives exist. Ketorolac has substantial asymptomatic GI effects.

Amiodarone is associated with QT interval problems and risks of provoking thyroid disease and declines in pulmonary function, while lacking sufficient evidence of benefit in older adults. Orphenadrine causes more sedation and anticholinergic adverse effects than safer alternatives in seniors.

Guanethidine and guanadrel both cause orthostatic hypotension and have safer alternatives. Isoxsuprine has not been shown to be effective in older adults. Nitrofurantoin has potential for renal impairment and safer options in seniors. Doxazosin can cause hypotension, dry mouth, and urinary incontinence. Methyltestosterone has the potential for prostatic hypertrophy and cardiac problems in seniors.

Thioridazine has a greater potential for CNS and extra parameatal effects than other antipsychotics. Mesoridazine also has CNS and extraparameatal adverse effects. Short-acting nifedipine can cause hypotension as well as constipation and edema.

Clonidine has been linked to orthostatic hypotension. Mineral oil has a potential for aspiration and adverse events associated with that. It is better to use safer alternatives that are available. Cimetidine is generally avoided because of CNS adverse events including confusion overall.

Ethacrynic acid has the potential for hypertension and fluid electrolyte imbalances with other safer options available. Desiccated thyroid is generally avoided in older adults due to concerns about cardiac effects with safer, more controlled dosing of other agents available. Estrogens also were on the list due to the evidence of breast and endometrial carcinogenicity and the lack of any cardiac protective effect in older adults.

Polypharmacy and Drug Burden

Not only are specific drugs problematic for older adults, but simply increasing the number of drugs taken increases the risk for adverse events among seniors, even more so than among younger adults [2, 3]. Hence, it is not adequate to simply avoid certain medications, but a constant effort to identify opportunities to debride medications from the medication list is needed.

The greater the number of medications, then the greater will be the difficulty with compliance. The more complex the medication regimen, the more likely that doses will be missed. Cost of medications also becomes a factor. If a drug is not on formulary, if the copay is too high, if the Part D Medicare benefit is tapped for the year, there is a greater likelihood that the prescription will not be filled or will be taken sporadically. All of these factors combined with the increases in comorbidity and aging itself make the senior population the most challenging of all when considering prescription medications. Any chance to simplify the medication regimen must be taken. Drugs that may have been useful when someone was younger may no longer be necessary. For example, if orthostatic hypotension develops, it may be time to reduce or eliminate an antihypertensive. Given the excessive risk for morbidity and mortality among those with orthostasis, hypertension might actually be the lesser of two evils. Certainly, when someone enters hospice, the bisphosphonates are probably no longer necessary in the treatment of osteoporosis, since most will remain stable for a longer period than the anticipated survival. Such efforts to reduce medication burden are always reasonable and vigilance for such opportunities should be a mainstay of geriatrics care.

Conclusion

The Beers criteria give some reasonable guidance for the identification of drugs to be avoided in seniors. Other drugs that have not made the list also may be candidates. Clinical circumstances as well as others may also be factors in deciding when to discontinue or adjust medications. Keeping the regimen as simple as possible should help with compliance and improve medication management overall, especially in a population of frail seniors.

References

1. Fick DM, Cooper JW, Wade WE et al (2003) Updating the Beers criteria for potentially inappropriate medication use in older adults. Arch Intern Med 163:2716–2724
2. Karas S (1981) The potential for drug interactions. Ann Emerg Med 10:627–630
3. Mühlberg W, Platt D (1999) Age-dependent changes of the kidneys: pharmacological implications. Gerontology 45:243–253

Dosing Errors: Age-Related Changes in Pharmacokinetics

Andrew J. McLachlan, Sarah N. Hilmer, and David G. Le Couteur

Keywords Older people • Elderly • Ageing • Geriatric pharmacology • Pharmacokinetics • Pharmacodynamics • Drug metabolism • Frailty

Pharmacological Basis of Pharmacotherapy

All substances are poisons; there is none which is not a poison. The right dose differentiates a poison from a remedy

Phillipus Aureolus Theophrastus Bombastas Von Hohenheim Paracelsus (sixteenth century)

The quality use of medicines focuses on using medicines safely and effectively once the right medicine is selected for the right patient. As Paracelsus identified, dose is a critical factor in ensuring that a patient receives benefit from a medicine with an acceptably low risk of unwanted side effects. The choice of the *right* dose for the *right* patient to achieve the *right* response is ultimately linked to a detailed understanding of the pharmacokinetics (relationship between dose, concentration and time) and pharmacodynamics (concentration–effect relationship) of a drug (Fig. 1) in the patient of interest. The relationship between the dose of a medicine that is administered and the patient response is a complex interplay of a number of competing events (Fig. 1). Once a drug is administered orally, it must leave the dose form (disintegrate) and dissolve into solution (dissolution) prior to being absorbed in the gastrointestinal tract. When the drug reaches the systemic circulation, it may bind to circulating plasma proteins, distribute and bind to tissue sites, be biotransformed to metabolites by organs such as the liver, be eliminated by the kidney or

A.J. McLachlan (✉)
Faculty of Pharmacy, University of Sydney, Sydney, NSW, Australia
and
Centre for Education and Research on Ageing, Concord Repatriation General Hospital, Hospital Road, Concord, NSW 2139, Australia
e-mail: andrew.mclachlan@sydney.edu.au

S. Koch et al. (eds.), *Medication Management in Older Adults:*
A Concise Guide for Clinicians, DOI 10.1007/978-1-60327-457-9_12,
© Springer Science+Business Media, LLC 2010

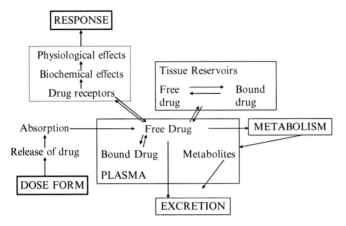

Fig. 1 Drug action and disposition

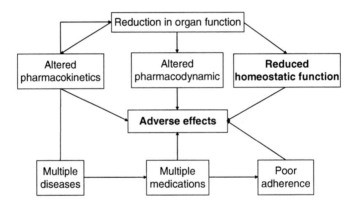

Fig. 2 Understanding adverse effects in older people

excreted in bile, and a portion will reach the site of action to interact with the response elements and alter a physiological process leading to the desired pharmacological response (Fig. 1).

Changes in any of these pharmacokinetic processes can therefore have an impact on the ability of the drug to access the site of action and ultimately illicit its pharmacological actions. It is clear that the interpatient variability in pharmacokinetic and pharmacodynamic processes contributes to the variability in drug response and contributes to the risk of the adverse effects (Fig. 2).

This chapter provides a commentary on the age-associated changes that occur in drug and metabolite pharmacokinetics in older people. The impact of ageing on the pharmacokinetics and pharmacodynamics of medicines has already been reviewed extensively [1–7]. It is important to note that while this chapter will focus primarily on aspects of the absorption, distribution, metabolism and excretion of drugs, this information must be considered in the context of the concentration–effect relationship for drugs and metabolites.

The Right Dose for the Right Older Person

The pharmacological basis of drug action implies that pharmacokinetics and pharmacodynamics of a drug are central to selecting the optimal dose; however, in reality, the selection of a drug and dose regimen for a patient is multifactorial. Dosing recommendations are formulated and refined based on the evidence from controlled clinical trials. However, in the case of older people, clinical trial data is often lacking to inform the quality use of medicines. For example, a review by Nair [8] found that only 3% of randomised, controlled trials and 1% of published meta-analyses include people over 65 years. More recently, Ridda et al. [9] highlight that frail older people are systematically excluded from clinical trials despite the fact that older people represent a considerable portion of people taking medicines in our community and arguably stand to gain the most from strong evidence to support appropriate drug and dose choice. This poses significant challenges to clinicians in accessing evidence that can inform practice and in particular dose regimen choice. Yet, Ridda et al. [9] demonstrate that conducting trials with frail older people is feasible by recruiting 300 older frail to a clinical study.

The clinical dilemma of choosing the right dose for the right older patient then comes from a balance between clinical evidence (which is lacking) and pharmacological principles. This implies that clinicians can utilise information about the known pharmacological properties of a drug, considering the factors that influence the pharmacokinetics and pharmacodynamics of the medicine and interpret these in the context of an individual's clinical status and characteristics to select an appropriate dosing and monitoring regimen.

The following sections provide a commentary on the impact of ageing on the four fates of a drug – absorption, distribution, metabolism and excretion. The effects of the age-related changes in pharmacokinetics on dosing are summarised in Table 1.

Absorption and Older People

Clinical data from a range of sources highlight changes in the gastrointestinal tract associated with ageing such as increased gastric pH, delayed gastric emptying, reduced gastrointestinal motility and intestinal blood flow [3, 10, 11]. The extent of age-associated changes in the gastrointestinal tract is highly variable [11]. However, these changes do not seem to have a significant effect on the extent of drug absorption and if anything may subtly slow the rate of absorption [3, 5, 6, 10]. One key observation is that the age-associated decline in intrinsic drug metabolic activity and liver blood flow has the potential to result in a decreased first-pass effect of some drugs causing

Table 1 Age-associated changes in pharmacokinetics: implications for dosing in older patients

Pharmacokinetic factor	Age-associated change	Implication for dosing	Example
Absorption	Complete but slower	Overall not significant	
Distribution	Reduced lean muscle mass, increased fat mass	Adjust loading dose to volume of distribution	Digoxin loading dose reduced by 15%
Metabolism	Decreased	Less first pass metabolism increases oral bioavailability Reduce maintenance dose of hepatically cleared drugs	Nitrates Morphine Propranolol Verapamil
Elimination	Decreased renal function common	Reduce maintenance dose of renally excreted drugs according to creatinine clearance	Enoxaparin Aminoglycosides

an increase in the systemic exposure [3]. This is one contributing factor to the excessive effects associated with orally administered nitrates observed in some older people [33]. Achlorhydria can occur in older people (either via age-associated changes [11] or the wide spread use of proton pump inhibitors), which can impair the absorption of medicines such as poorly soluble weak bases like dipyridamole [13]. Russell et al. [13] demonstrated that dipyridamole bioavailability was pH-sensitive in older people such that achlorhydrics had considerable lower and variable drug absorption. In the acute aged care setting, people are more likely to experience swallowing difficulties [14], which leads to changes in the manner in which a medicine is administered or dose form modification (see Chap. 4).

The possible effects of ageing on the absorption of medicines from slow release formulations have not been systematically studied. One common route of administration in this clinical setting, which has the potential to alter the drug absorption process, is administration via nasogastric tube. For example, a study by Kotake et al. [15] indicated that bioavailability of medicines, such as amiodarone, are significantly reduced when administered by nasogastric tube. This has important implications, and care should be taken when switching routes of administration in this manner to carefully monitor patients for lack of clinical efficacy and potential toxicity.

Distribution

Ageing is associated with changes in body composition, with an increase in body fat (from 18 to 36% in men and from 33to 45% in women) and approximately 10% decrease in body water [16]. The increase in the proportion of body fat may be related to a decline in total body weight at the expense of lean body weight [10, 17, 18]. This is likely to result in a larger volume of distribution and, hence, longer half-life of lipophilic drugs and a higher plasma concentration of hydrophilic drugs. The decline in the proportion of lean body weight has been associated with a decline in the volume of distribution of digoxin, which binds to the NaKATPase in skeletal muscle [19]. The clinical impact of these changes in volume of distribution on digoxin dose regimen design is uncertain, given the age-associated decline in renal function (primarily route of elimination) for digoxin [20]. Human serum albumin concentrations also decline with age [21, 22], which has important implications for the distribution and hepatic metabolism of some highly bound drugs and metabolites.

However, the overall effect on pharmacokinetics and therefore maintenance dose requirements needs to be considered in the light of the possible effect that altered unbound concentration might have on the hepatic and renal clearance. Loading doses (i.e. the first dose given to a person to achieve therapeutic concentrations) in older people need to be adjusted according the age-associated effect on a drug's volume of distribution. For example, in frail older people, who have a lower volume of distribution, require a lower loading dose of digoxin [19]. In summary, age-associated changes in body composition are not always clinically significant and thus do not universally result in dose regimen alterations [3].

Drug Metabolism in Older Age

Until recently, the information regarding the impact of ageing of drug metabolism has been confusing and conflicting [3, 23]. What is clear is that physiological parameters that are likely to impact on a person's ability to metabolise medicines are altered – for example, there is an age-associated decline in both liver size and hepatic blood flow [3, 10, 23]. Sotaniemi et al. [24] investigated the cytochrome P450 (CYP) content in liver biopsy samples and antipyrine clearance after oral administration in 226 people and found that both CYP content and drug metabolising activity decline with age. Whereas, Schwartz [25] found that drug metabolism activity (as assessed using the erythromycin breath test) actually appeared to increase in older frail people. More recently, an insightful reanalysis by Butler and Begg [26] reminded us that hepatic clearance of a drug or metabolite is a function of the intrinsic metabolic activity of the liver, fraction unbound and hepatic blood flow. These authors carefully considered the available data for medicines, which have capacity-limited metabolism (or low hepatic extraction ratios) where intrinsic metabolic activity and protein binding are highly influential. When the unbound hepatic clearance for highly bound capacity-limited medicines (such as naproxen, valproic acid, ibuprofen, oxaprozin, temazepam, lorazepam, diazepam, phenytoin and warfarin) was estimated, there is compelling evidence of an age-associated decrease in drug metabolic activity [26]. Furthermore, these authors [26] highlight that few pharmacokinetic studies in older people measure the fraction unbound and that this should be a key consideration in pharmacokinetic calculations.

A key factor that can affect a person's ability to metabolise a medicine relates to the concomitant drug therapy and the risk of drug–drug interactions that can cause inhibition or induction of drug metabolism [2, 3, 23, 27]. Polypharmacy in older people is major concern and a significant risk factor for adverse effects and drug–drug interactions [3, 4]. A recent study by Tulner et al. [27] highlighted the high prevalence and variable significance of drug–drug interactions in an outpatient population of older people. In this study, almost half of the older outpatients (mean age 81 years; $n = 807$) had potentially serious drug–drug interactions identified, and a quarter of these patients were experiencing possible adverse events or reduced effectiveness of medicines that may have been at least in part contributed by these interactions [27].

The age-associated changes in drug pharmacokinetics (commonly leading to higher systemic exposure at regular doses) pose a significant risk for metabolic interactions by substrate inhibition, the clinical significance of which are con-centration-dependent. This clearly has implications for both commencing new medicines for new indications for older person and ceasing medicines [3, 23]. Gorski et al. [28] examined the impact of age (younger and older) on metabolic induction interactions (using rifampicin to induce midazolam metabolism by CYP3A4). These authors found that age did not influence the extent of induction in this case.

Elimination

While it is generally accepted (and taught) that renal function declines as a person ages [6], the extent of renal impairment is highly variable in older people [3, 10]. Sitar [10] has highlighted that data from longitudinal studies suggest that age-associated decline in renal function is not universal and one-third of patients seem to experience no significant decline in kidney function. This highlights the importance of individu-alising the dose of renally excreted medicines based on an individual's estimated renal function. Interestingly, there has been an expanding use of the MDRD equation (based on serum creatinine, age and ethnicity) to estimate a person's glomerular filtration rate – replacing creatinine clearance estimated using the Cockcroft and Gault formula – to adjustment of patient doses. However, the MDRD formula was designed as a screening tool to identify people with chronic kidney disease [29] and has not been directly correlated with drug renal clearance.

Roberts [30] compared the use of the Cockcroft and Gault formula to the MDRD formula in 1,067 older patients and found that the MDRD formula sig-nificantly overestimated renal function and would have led to significantly higher doses of enoxaparin and gentamicin (both of which rely predominately on renal excretion). This study highlights the need for further research to rigorously char-acterise the relationship between MDRD estimates of renal function and drug clearance before this formula can be recommended to guide dose adjustment in the clinical setting.

Frailty and Pharmacokinetics

Chronological age itself is not a reliable determinant of a drug's pharmacokinetic behaviour [1–7]. A number of studies have examined the impact of frailty as an independent predictor of pharmacokinetic response [25, 31, 32]. Frailty is characterised by a decline in physiological reserve and includes, among other characteristics, sarcopenia [12] which could theoretically impact on drug distribution, but only a few studies have attempted to assess the impact of frailty on pharmacokinetics and drug dosing.

As discussed, Schwartz [25] investigated the hypothesis that frailty, independently of age, maybe an important factor in determining drug elimination capacity by using the erythromycin breath test as a marker of metabolic activity. It was concluded that old and very old (>80 years) people maintain the ability to metabolise drugs via some metabolic pathways and frail people do not display reduced drug clearance via these pathways. The impact of frailty on metoclopramide sulphation has been studied and it was found that the activity of this pathway is preserved in otherwise fit older subjects, but is significantly decreased in frail older people. In a separate study, Wynne et al. [31] [32] also investigated the effects of frailty on paracetamol glucuronidation confirming that frailty was more influential than age alone. Taken together, these results suggest frailty has a global effect on conjugation pathways. What is clear from the available studies is that the pharmacokinetics of medicines in frail older people are poorly understood. Given the diminished reserve in these patients, they are at greater risk of adverse effects from medicines (Fig. 2). There is a lack of high quality evidence and the available information is often conflicting. Studies to establish the impact of frailty on other pharmacokinetic parameters are needed to inform dose regimen design in this cohort of older people.

Start Low, Go Slow

This mantra of medical education has become the universal recommendation for dosing in older people. While this seems a reasonable and justifiable approach, which has a focus on minimising the risk of possible adverse effects, it has the potential to lead to undertreatment. For example, when treating a serious bacterial infection starting antibiotic doses "low" and increasing the dose "slowly" is irrational leading to the risk of inadequate antimicrobial treatment, the development of resistance and poor clinical outcome. A similar scenario may play out in the case of "starting low and going slow" with analgesics. Inadequate pain relief may lead to the escalation of medicine choice with a person receiving opioids when simple analgesics – used at adequate doses – may be clinically appropriate. The choice of the starting dose regimen is a critical step that can be informed by knowledge of the pharmacokinetics and pharmacodynamics of a medicine in older people. Quality use of medicines demands that once a dose regimen is selected the patient receives ongoing monitoring to adjust the dose to ensure optimal patient outcomes.

Conclusion

The principles of pharmacokinetics and pharmacodynamics are important considerations in providing information on the optimal dose of a medicine in the absence of clinical evidence from rigorous clinical trials in the patient group of interest. The individualisation of dosing regimens should not be based solely on chronological age but should account for age-associated changes in a drug's pharmacokinetics and pharmacodynamics.

References

1. Abernethy DR (1999) Aging effects on drug disposition and effect. Geriatr Nephrol Urol 9:15–19
2. Hilmer SN, McLachlan A, Le Couteur DG (2007) Clinical pharmacology in geriatric patients. Fundam Clin Pharmacol 21:217–230
3. McLean AJ, Le Couteur DG (2004) Aging biology and geriatric clinical pharmacology. Pharmacol Rev 56:163–184
4. Le Couteur DG, Hilmer SN, Glasgow N, Naganathan V, Cumming RG (2004) Prescribing in older people. Aust Fam Physician 33:777–781
5. Turnheim K (2003) When drug therapy gets old: pharmacokinetics and pharmacodynamics in the elderly. Exp Gerontol 38(8):843–853
6. Cusack BJ (2004) Pharmacokinetics in older persons. Am J Geriatr Pharmacother 2:274–302
7. Hammerlein A, Derendorf H, Lowenthal DT (1998) Pharmacokinetic and pharmacodynamic changes in the elderly: clinical implications. Clin Pharmacokinet 35:49–64
8. Nair BR (2002) Evidence based medicine for older people: available, accessible, acceptable, adaptable? Aust J Ageing 21:58–60
9. Ridda I, Lindley R, MacIntyre RC (2008) The challenges of clinical trials in the exclusion zone: the case of the frail elderly. Australas J Ageing 27:61–66
10. Sitar DS (2007) Aging issues in drug disposition and efficacy. Proc West Pharmacol Soc 50:16–20
11. Bhutto A, Morley JE (2008) The clinical significance of gastrointestinal changes with aging. Curr Opin Clin Nutr Metab Care 11:651–660
12. Fried LP, Tangen CM, Walston J, Newman AB, Hirsch C, Gottdiener J, Seeman T, Tracy R, Kop WJ, Burke G, McBurnie MA, Cardiovascular Health Study Collaborative Research Group (2001) Frailty in older adults: evidence for a phenotype. J Gerontol A Biol Sci Med Sci 56:M146–M156
13. Russell TL, Berardi RR, Barnett JL, O'Sullivan TL, Wagner JG, Dressman JB (1994) pH-related changes in the absorption of dipyridamole in the elderly. Pharm Res 11:136–143
14. Stubbs J, Haw C, Dickens G (2008) Dose form modification – a common but potentially hazardous practice. A literature review and study of medication administration to older psychiatric inpatients. Int Psychogeriatr 20:616–627
15. Kotake T, Takada M, Goto T, Komamura K, Kamakura S, Morishita H (2006) Serum amiodarone and desethylamiodarone concentrations following nasogastric versus oral administration. J Clin Pharm Ther 31:237–243
16. Vestal RE (1997) Aging and pharmacology. Cancer 80:1302–1310
17. Kyle UG, Genton L, Hans D, Karsegard L, Slosman DO, Pichard C (2001) Age-related differences in fat-free mass, skeletal muscle, body cell mass and fat mass between 18 and 94 years. Eur J Clin Nutr 55(8):663–672
18. Newman AB, Lee JS, Visser M, Goodpaster BH, Kritchevsky SB, Tylavsky FA, Nevitt M, Harris TB (2005) Weight change and the conservation of lean mass in old age: the Health, Aging and Body Composition Study. Am J Clin Nutr 82:872–878

19. Hanratty CG, McGlinchey P, Johnston GD et al (2000) Differential pharmacokinetics of digoxin in elderly patients. Drugs Aging 17:353–362
20. Miura T, Kojima R, Sugiura Y et al (2000) Effect of aging on the incidence of digoxin toxicity. Ann Pharmacother 34:427–432
21. Salive ME, Cornoni-Huntley J, Phillips CL, Guralnik JM, Cohen HJ, Ostfeld AM, Wallace RB (1992) Serum albumin in older persons: relationship with age and health status. J Clin Epidemiol 45:213–221
22. Visser M, Kritchevsky SB, Newman AB, Goodpaster BH, Tylavsky FA, Nevitt MC, Harris TB (2005) Lower serum albumin concentration and change in muscle mass: the Health, Aging and Body Composition Study. Am J Clin Nutr 82:531–537
23. Wynne H (2005) Drug metabolism and ageing. J Br Menopause Soc 11:51–56
24. Sotaniemi EA, Arranto AJ, Pelkonen O, Pasanen M (1997) Age and cytochrome P450-linked drug metabolism in humans: an analysis of 226 subjects with equal histopathologic conditions. Clin Pharmacol Ther 61:331–339
25. Schwartz JB (2006) Erythromycin breath test results in elderly, very elderly, and frail elderly persons. Clin Pharmacol Ther 79:440–448
26. Butler JM, Begg EJ (2008) Free drug metabolic clearance in elderly people. Clin Pharmacokinet 47:297–321
27. Tulner LR, Frankfort SV, Gijsen GJ, van Campen JP, Koks CH, Beijnen JH (2008) Drug-drug interactions in a geriatric outpatient cohort: prevalence and relevance. Drugs Aging 25:343–355
28. Gorski JC, Vannaprasaht S, Hamman MA, Ambrosius WT, Bruce MA, Haehner-Daniels B, Hall SD (2003) The effect of age, sex and rifampicin administration on intestinal and hepatic cytochrome P4503A activity. Clin Pharmacol Ther 74:275–287
29. Mathew TH, Johnson DW, Jones GRD on behalf of the Australasian Creatinine Consensus Working Group (2007) Chronic kidney disease and automatic reporting of estimated glomerular filtration rate: revised recommendations. Med J Aust 187:459–463
30. Roberts GW (2006) Dosing of key renally cleared drugs in the elderly-time to be wary of the eGFR. J Pharm Prac Res 3:204–209
31. Wynne HA, Cope LH, Herd B, Rawlins MD, James OF, Woodhouse KW (1990) The association of age and frailty with paracetamol conjugation in man. Age Ageing 19:419–424
32. Wynne HA, Yelland C, Cope LH, Boddy A, Woodhouse KW, Bateman DN (1993) The association of age and frailty with the pharmacokinetics and pharmacodynamics of metoclopramide. Age Ageing 22:354–359
33. Kelly JG, O'Malley K (1992) Nitrates in the elderly. Pharmacological considerations. Drugs Aging 2:14–19

Index